CULTURAL LANGUAGE DIFFERENCES

CULTURAL LANGUAGE DIFFERENCES

Their Educational and Clinical-Professional Implications

Edited by

SOL ADLER, Ph.D.

Professor and Director
Pediatric Language Programs
Department of Audiology and Speech Pathology
University of Tennessee
Knoxville, Tennessee

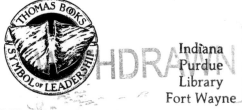

CHARLES C THOMAS • PUBLISHER
Springfield • Illinois • U.S.A.

Published and Distributed Throughout the World by

CHARLES C THOMAS • PUBLISHER

2600 South First Street

Springfield, Illinois 62717

© *1984 by* CHARLES C THOMAS • PUBLISHER

ISBN 0-398-05030-9

Library of Congress Catalog Card Number: 84-2538

With THOMAS BOOKS *careful attention is given to all details of manufacturing and
design. It is the Publisher's desire to present books that are satisfactory as to their physical
qualities and artistic possibilities and appropriate for their particular use.* THOMAS
BOOKS *will be true to those laws of quality that assure a good name and good will.*

Printed in the United States of America
Q-R-3

Library of Congress Cataloging in Publication Data
Main entry under title:

Cultural language differences.

Bibliography: p.
1. Speech and social status--United States--Addresses,
essays, lectures.   2. Language arts--United States--
Remedial teaching--Addresses essays, lectures.   3. Speech
therapy for children--United States--Addresses, essays,
lectures.   4. English language--Study and teaching
(Elementary)--United States--Addresses, essays, lectures.
I. Adler, Sol, 1925-
P40.5.S63C85   1984   40'.9'0973   84-2538
ISBN 0-398-05030-9

CONTRIBUTORS

KENDALL BERGIN
Doctoral Student
Department of Audiology and Speech Pathology
University of Tennessee
Knoxville, Tennessee

NICHOLAS BOUNTRESS, PH.D.
Associate Professor
Department of Communicative Disorders
Old Dominion University
Norfolk, Virginia

SANDRA L. TERRELL, PH.D.
Assistant Professor
Division of Communication Disorders
North Texas State University
Denton, Texas

BETHEL H. WOMACK
Graduate Student
Department of Audiology and Speech Pathology
University of Tennessee
Knoxville, Tennessee

PREFACE

THIS book of essays is a compilation of articles that are relevant to cultural language differences and their educational and clinical implications. The book is addressed mainly to speech-language clinicians and educators, but it is of obvious pertinence to all professional workers who interact with children, adolescents, or adults who happen to speak a social dialect.

We believe there is a need for bidialectal-bicultural training programs for speakers of social dialects; we support the idea that such training should be initiated in preschool programs but is also effective when taught in elementary, high school, or college. Moreover, wherever social dialect speakers congregate in a learning environment, such training should be a part of the educational program provided for them.

None of the recent reports emanating from the Federal Government or Foundations concerning the inadequacy of our schools address the problem of *unequal* education between the middle and lower-classes; that it is the poor and lower-class children who are performing most inadequately in our schools.

We believe that speech-language clinicians, should, as one of their job descriptions, try to convince educators to implement bidialectal and bicultural programs: to provide them not only with the knowledge undergirding bidialectalism but also the means — the lesson plans — to develop such programs.

Such information, and much more, is provided in this book. We hope the book will serve to alert these workers to the theme we enunciated in a previous book (*Poverty Children and Their Language*), that current teaching-treating strategies are simply not effective for poor children who speak a social dialect. We must transcend the conventional and implement innovative bidialectal programs in the schools and the clinics.

INTRODUCTION

THIS book addresses clinical issues in two environments: the schools and the clinics. The professional implications of these issues are particularly relevant to the Speech-Language Pathologist (SLP).* They are also important to school teachers, psychologists, special educators, remedial reading specialists, and indeed any professional worker who interacts with culturally-different and poor children.

It is the children— children who speak a social dialect — whom we are particularly concerned about. It is our belief that many of these children (as well as adolescents and adults) suffer from inappropriate teaching-treating strategies that negatively influence their future.

In the Schools

Current and conventional teaching strategies are inadequate for poor children who simply are not learning appropriate educational skills. There is need for a new approach — a new teaching strategy — to obviate these educational problems. We believe there is a need for bidialectal-bicultural training programs in our schools, particularly preschool and K-2 grades. The intent of this book, in part, is to demonstrate the need and propriety for such programming, as well as its effectiveness. If social dialects such as Black and Appalachian

---

*We use the labels "speech-language clinician" and "speech-language pathologist" interchangeably throughout the book.

ix

English† are rule-governed, as research demonstrates they are, these dialects should be retained — as foreign languages are retained by immigrants to this country.

Due to social and political reasons, as we point out in one of our essays, little has been done to implement such programs. People find it difficult to accept these social dialect patterns as nonstandard linguistic differences, instead of substandard speech-language deficiencies.

In Part I, "Social Dialects in Our Schools," proficiency testing clearly demonstrates that educational failure is rooted in the lower socio-economic classes — not because of traditional reasons (i.e., insufficiency of parental support, help, and stimulation, or simply the impoverished environment, although all may be relevant), but rather the result of dialectal and cultural conflicts that exist in the schools. The interrelationship between talking in a social dialect and its impact upon reading and particularly writing skills is discussed in a report by Kendall Bergin. "The Relationship of English Composition Grades to Oral (Social) Dialect: An Analysis of Dialectal and Non-Dialectal Writing Errors," demonstrates clearly the need to teach oral standard English skills in English composition classes.

Clinical and Professional Implications

Nicholas Bountress in his chapter "Social Dialects and the Speech-Language Clinician: An Overview of Clinical and Professional Issues" presents to the reader the various issues and problems surrounding the social dialect speaker in his/her interaction with professional workers. The article by myself and coauthor I.A. Whitman Tims, "The Pediatric Language Specialist: An Innovative Approach to Early Language Intervention and the Role of the Speech-Language Clinician," expands upon some of the issues raised by Bountress. Sandra Terrell's contribution "Issues in Layperson Bias Toward the Cultural Difference View," points out very convincingly the impact social dialects have upon American auditors. Lastly, Beth Womack, in "Language Intervention in the School and

---

†In this book we stress the implications to Black English and Appalachian English speakers; other speakers of dialects such as "Mex-Tex" (Hispanic English as spoken in the Southwestern part of our country) have similar problems, and the matters discussed in this book are of obvious relevance to them.

in the Clinic: The Role of the Speech-Language Pathologist in School and Non-School Environments," stresses the dynamics involved in the implementation of a program that is both relevant and fair to the dialect speaker. Ms. Womack, a practicing Speech-Language Clinician in a rural Appalachian school system, addresses these matters in a pragmatic and realistic manner.

The Establishment Dialect and Mores

Our democracy presupposes social class mobility, that is, the opportunity for all to pull themselves up the social class ladder to a better way of life. For lower-class people to move up the ladder, and to be accepted by middle class establishment society, the ability to talk and behave as do inhabitants of the establishment society is required. It is therefore incumbent upon educators to furnish all children with the standard dialect and mores, since it is readily observable that these skills are not being provided to lower-class children. By not furnishing these skills educators detract from the democratic ideal. That the acceptance of lower-class and minority peoples into the establishment mainstream is negatively affected by factors other than speech-language dialect and behavioral mores is well known; for example the insidious effect of racism that permeates our society is clearly of fundamental inportance. Yet the significance of the negative attitude exhibited by middle-class auditory towards lower-class dialects and mores is also of much importance and should not be ignored. For example, see the study by Terrell in Part II of this book that documents the pejorative impact of Black English upon middle class auditors.

To continue to ignore the deleterious impact that social dialect patterns may have on its possessor is unconscionable. As discussed in detail in this book, there are three methods being used to "treat" the dialect.

Those people who argue for the continued and indeed the extended use of the eradicationist teaching technique and philosophy, whereby social dialect patterns are eliminated, are simply ignoring the reality of the situation — it does not work. Those protagonists of the non-intervention or "laissez faire" philosophy, whereby nothing is done about the dialect, are also ignoring reality — non-interventionism does not allow for upward class mobility for those who desire it. This book argues for the development of bidialectal and bicultural teaching-treating strategies. In our experiences, its utilization has been effective insofar as standard or establishment English development is concerned, and teachers who have used it under our guidance have been supportive of it.

We wish to thank the other contributors to the book; we hope they will be pleased with the finished product.

Contents

xiii

CULTURAL LANGUAGE
DIFFERENCES

Part I

EDUCATIONAL IMPLICATIONS

Chapter I

ILLITERACY IN OUR SCHOOLS

An Introduction

SOL ADLER

Educational Retardation

A PBS television presentation in 1982 indicated a *scandal exists* (their terminology) in our American public schools: it was indicated that the illiteracy rate among poor children is very high and that the rate is increasing rather than decreasing; by illiteracy they referred mainly to a severe depression in reading skills. During a relatively recent California I.Q. court case, for example, it was noted that many poor black high school students were reading at approximately a third grade level, and that there was much educational retardation in this population of adolescents.*

This condition is not new. In the early 1960's when the war on poverty was initiated, Head-Start and subsequently Title I compensatory education programs were developed to attenuate the educational retardation found in poor children. This compensatory philosophy is rooted in both the experiential and the cognitive-language differences of poor children. To compensate for these diferences the children are exposed to middle-class experiences, their parents are counseled regarding the development of a home environ-

---

*Larry P.vs. Riles, 1979.

ment conducive to educational acquisition, and intensive cognitive-language training programs are developed for the children.

Although all of these strategies are useful, they have not obviated the educational failure manifested by poor children. The children still show inferior academic skills as noted on proficiency test scores administered in almost any city in the country.

Proficiency Tests & Educational Retardation

Proficiency tests are a relatively recent occurrence on the educational scene. Their advent is related to the recognition that educational retardation among the poor continues to be a significant and serious problem confronting our school systems. In many states using proficiency tests, the ninth grade has been chosen as the academic cut-off point; that is, all ninth graders must take this test and demonstrate certain grade level of proficiency if they are to be allowed to eventually graduate from high school and receive a diploma. Those students unable to demonstrate this level of competence are usually given other chances. If they are still unable to obtain the requisite scores, they are allowed to complete their education and receive a document indicating they have completed 12 years of schooling — but they do not receive a diploma. However, the granting of a diploma does not guarantee literacy. In some states apparently only a fourth grade reading level is required to pass the test.

Analysis of the proficiency test scores will reveal that lower-class (poor) children score on a significantly lower level than do their more affluent peers; that the few middle-class children who fail the proficiency reading test probably possess a learning disability — a dyslexia. When one analyzes the failure rate it can be seen that a higher percentage of poor black children fail the test than their white peers. In the state of Tennessee, for example, the cosmopolitan cities of Memphis, Nashville, and Knoxville demonstrated higher failure rates than did their respective counties. One reason for this discrepancy between county and city failure rates resides in the higher number of poor black children who live in the cities.

Reasons Cited for the Educational Failure

Some people believe that the educational failure manifested by poor children is due to a genetic and intellectual inferiority (see for example, Professor Hernnstein's article in the August 1982 issue of *The Atlantic Monthly,* "I.Q. Testing and the Media"). Others, particularly educators, claim it is related to an unresponsive and uncaring home environment. The nature vs. nurture controversy. We do not accept the validity of the former theory and we believe the environmental cause has been exaggerated. There are a variety of reasons for this: (1) the lower-class is not homogenous, it is comprised of both upper-lower and lower-lower-classes. The former class generally contains an organized and stable family environment concerned about the childrens' educational welfare. (2) The presence in the home of books or other reading material, the lack of which is frequently claimed to be related to educational failure, is no guarantee that the children will receive superior stimulation in the home. The books must be read before they can enhance learning. (3) Lastly, as citizens, the children of the lower-class poor simply deserve a better education than they currently receive, regardless of problems in the home environment. The fault resides we think, not with the child, his family or teacher, but with the teaching philosophies that are currently being utilized.

It is our contention that the root cause of this problem is the cultural and dialectal conflicts which occur in the classroom. These conflicts are not obviated, but are often enhanced, by the classroom teacher. This is particularly the case with white teachers and black children. The mores, values, behaviors — including linguistic and paralinguistic (body language and speech prosody) behaviors — of poor black children are generally alien to middle-class white teachers. It is this conflict in cultural patterns that creates much of the motivational and linguistic problems in these children.

Teachers generally react to language patterns that are not acceptable to their middle-class cultural standards by using either the eradication or the non-intervention response. In the former they try to eliminate or eradicate the social dialect utterance, overtly by telling the child that his or her linguistic utterance is inappropriate, or covertly by repeating what the child said in the standard English model. The non-intervention technique entails the acceptance of the utterance without any attempt to change it. Both teaching strategies are ineffective or inappropriate: the former has not generally succeeded in teaching the child standard English or middle-class behavioral patterns — it is an ineffective strategy; and the latter, by accepting the child's utterances or behaviors, is inappropriate because it does not equip the child to perform adequately in the middle-class classroom or in the middle-class job market.

Historically, two problems occur to speakers of lower-class social dialects: a history of educational retardation and a history of failure in the job market for the high school or college graduate. Both of these problems are related to the speakers inability to speak in standard English and to manifest middle-class behavior patterns. Both reading and writing skills taught to children in the lower grades necessitate an understanding of standard English grammatical rules and lexicon. Those children who enter the early grades talking in a social dialect, particularly black English, will experience much difficulty in learning the standard English reading and writing skills being taught in these grades. Most early elementary school teachers will confirm this fact - that there is a correlation between severity of oral dialect and inteference with the acquisition of reading and writing skills. Some recent research completed at the College level reveals a similar correlation between severity of oral dialect and failure in Freshman English Composition classes. Black students who used much Black English in their speech patterns had a much higher rate of failure than did their black student peers who used much less Black English. (see the following chapter.)

There are also many examples of the limitation placed upon social dialect speakers when they enter the job market. The research clearly demonstrates that a negative attitude is held by middle-class listeners to speakers of social dialects. Many otherwise competent and intelligent people are unable to get responsible positions that they are eminently qualified to handle because of this negative stereotype. *

---

*According to a study by Terrell & Terrell, (*ASHA*, June 1983) black females who spoke Black English or standard English applied for vacant secretarial positions. Black English speakers were offered fewer jobs than standard English speakers. Additionally, the pay level for those positions offered to Black English speakers was significantly less than the pay offered to standard English speakers.

Similar findings were reported when a diglossic male, speaking in Black English was rejected for an interview by five prospective employers; when speaking in standard English he was granted an interview by the same employers (an article published by L. May, a reporter for the Sunday Magazine section of the Atlanta Journal & Constitution newspaper, June 24, 1979).

What To Do

It is obvious that speaking and behaving, in the middle-class manner, is necessary if the majority of lower class students are to achieve at their potential. This dictum is generally held to be true by most educators, yet little is being done to implement it. As previously stated, eradication teaching strategies are generally ineffective; for example, an examination of the speech patterns and behavioral mores of the poor students attending any high school located in the inner city or rural area will reveal that they possess much oral dialect and behavior patterns typical of their culture. The eradication method simply doesn't work, and the non-intervention strategy, is clearly self-defeating, doing nothing to prepare the student to enter the middle-class educational or job market.

We propose a bidialectal and bicultural teaching strategy. In this way, we truly integrate the schools by comparing and contrasting the linguistic and other cultural differences that exist in the desegregated schools. To ignore these differences, as is done in most desegregated schools, is to denegrate the cultural language and behavior patterns of poor children. In previous publications we have described how effective bidialectalism is in teaching standard English to culturally different children. Instead of eradicating the utterance by indicating to the child that his remarks were said incorrectly, we have used the term "Everyday Talk" as a label for his non-standard dialectal utterance, and the child is asked to compare and contrast it with "School Talk," the standard English equivalent. In this way, we legitimize his dialect — we recognize that such speech patterns are rule governed as is standard (we prefer the term establishment or network) English and differ only in prestige. We encourage the child to retain his cultural dialect and behavior but to develop the ability to switch — to become diglossic — as a function of the speech (or cultural) situation he is in . He is taught to use establishment English in school or in situations where such English patterns are expected, and to use social dialect in his home or everyday environment. It is the same idea that permeates bilingualism. When a teaching strategy is adopted in our schools which allows for the early development of bidialectal and bicultural skills, it may allow poor children to become literate (and motivated) members of our society.

Clearly, the educational strategies used in schools to educate the poor children, particularly poor black students, are generally ineffective. Proficiency tests confirm this. We must alter or change our teaching strategies so that these children can become literate and successful members of our society.

We believe the speech-language clinician must develop skills that will cater effectively to these needs; in brief they are:*

(1) Become familiar with the rules of the social dialects; be capable of distinguishing between speech-language deficiencies and differences.

(2) Develop testing and report-writing skills that are sensitive to cultural differences.

(3) Do not ignore linguistic differences in clinical programs; initiate a teaching program for those children possessing both deficiencies and differences.

(4) Be a consultant to teachers; help them to develop a bidialectal-bicultural teaching program.

---

*The September, 1983, issue of *Asha* addresses some of these issues in the Social Dialects section.

According to the September, 1983, *Asha* position paper on social dialects, such programming is elective. Thus, as noted in the most recent Student Evaluation Manual published by the Tennessee Department of Education, 1982 (pp. 11-15), when dialect differences are noted by the speech-language clinician, the differences " . . . are not to be considered as sufficient cause for accepting a child into speech therapy. They are . . . generally dealt with by the teacher in English class." We have underscored the fact however, that most teachers, be they English teachers or non-English teachers, are generally ineffective in their dealings with dialectal utterances. This problem is not unique to Tennessee; we believe that these dialectal patterns must be the ultimate responsibility of the speech-language clinician, either as a consultant to the teacher in the formulation of a bidialectal program and/or when addressing these dialect patterns in patients whom also possess substandard speech and are receiving treatment for their speech-language disorders.

The *Asha* paper on social dialects equivocates by indicating (1) the service to dialect speakers is elective, and (2) suggesting that either non-intervention or bidialectalism (without using this term) are acceptable intervention methods. The service should be mandatory and should entail a bidialectal teaching methodology.

Chapter II

SOCIAL DIALECTS AND LITERACY:

The Interrelation Among Talking, Reading, and Writing in Culturally Different and Poor Children

SOL ADLER

INEVITABLY, language plays a significant role in education and social acculturation. Used as a means of transmitting information, it is an essential ingredient in the development and utilization of educational skills and is a vehicle of social acceptance or non-acceptance, as people react to each other based on the way they speak. The importance of language in education, coupled with its social significance, makes it a key factor in the struggle for human equity.

Since the early 1960's, a great deal of research has been undertaken on language diversity in American English — particularly involving those groups who speak what has been labeled "non-standard" English, or social dialects. Research on these dialectal varieties has raised some fundamental educational and social issues — issues which must not be ignored by those vested with the responsibility of educating all students.

There are three major concerns relevant to the language of social

11

dialect speakers; that is, speakers of Black English, or Ebonics, and of Mountain or Appalachian English — our two major social dialects. First, there is a significant interrelationship between talking and reading/writing skill development, i.e., the attainment of literacy; because of this relationship, some speakers of social dialects often manifest poor academic skills. Second, the public's negative stereotypic perception of social dialect speakers causes many otherwise competent adults to have difficulty finding work appropriate to their skills. Third, there is a need for such speakers to learn to talk in standard or establishment English, but the strategies used to teach establishment English have generally been ineffective.

Clearly, we are generalizing. There are obviously some social dialect speakers who are very literate, possess good jobs, and who speak in their social dialect. But it is equally clear, we believe, that they are the exceptions to the rule. A greater number of social dialect speakers are both educationally and socially handicapped because of their dialect.

SOCIAL DIALECT SPEAKERS

As noted in the Ann Arbor decision by Federal Judge Charles Joiner (Bountress, 1980), one of the most significant problems facing children with reading problems who speak social dialects is the lack of their teachers' sensitivity to the dialect. Such insensitivity by teachers would appear to be related to the reading problems of children. Professional workers trained, respectively, in conventional language arts teaching and treating systems have, in general, inadequately helped these children to speak in standard English; standard English is simply not being used by the majority of minority-poor students. A function of the speech-language clinician is (1) to help teachers become sensitive to social dialects, and (2) to help them develop an effective bidialectal and bicultural teaching program (Adler, 1971a).

It seems appropriate to suggest that the Joiner decision may have an impact upon all social dialect speakers, ". . . that it is a precedent setting case" (Whiteman, 1980, P.V.) not only for those who speak Black English but also those who speak Mountain English as well; and not only in Ann Arbor, but in cities across the land.

The nonstandard or dialectal patterns of children are usually addressed by clinicians and educators by either the eradication or the acceptance (i.e., non-intervention) philosophies. Both have proven to be inadequate. The dialectal patterns are not being eradicated in the majority of culturally-different and poor students, and the acceptance of dialectal patterns is potentially harmful to the students' literacy and employment in certain occupations.

Clearly, it is time for teaching-treating strategies to be altered to take into account the implications of the Ann Arbor decision. If this does not occur, the courts may mandate that it be done.

THE PROBLEM

A casual survey in many of our elementary or high school hallways, as well as on college or university campuses, would reveal that economically poor students frequently speak a dialect relevant to their sociolinguistic heritage. Some of the children or adults will utilize only a minimal amount of dialect; others will use a significant amount. Some may use all linguistic and paralinguistic patterns associated with their social dialect; others may use standard (establishment) English linguistic patterns and nonstandard paralanguage (prosodic patterns and body language).

In particular, a sizable number of black students use nonstandard Black English dialect when talking. Similarly, we believe there is much Mountain (Appalachian) English dialect used in Appalachia or in the Midwest, where there are many emigrants from Appalachia. And, as suggested above, Black English, and Mountain English, are social dialects that may (1) impair the development of reading and writing skills, and (2) negatively affect employment opportunities.

We believe our profession has a responsibility to this population, many of whom possess excellent potential that may not be realized due, in part, to prejudicial attitudes towards such speakers.

The California I.Q. Case

Another landmark court case of relevance to minority poor children was the California litigation (C-71-2270; October 16, 1979) in which black children challenged the continued use of I.Q. tests as valid criteria for class placement — particularly E.M.R. class placement. Judge Peckham held that such tests had a disproportionate effect on black children.

During the discussion inherent to the decision, it was noted that black children: (1) learn about .7 as much as middle class white children; (2) fall increasingly behind in their educational development ". . . to the point that it is not unusual for High School Students to be reading at the third grade level" (p. 932). It was also noted that ". . . there are a very great many studies in which the socioeconomic status indices have been held constant. The almost uniform finding is that the blacks still score lower than the whites" (p. 956). ". . . It is essential that California's educators confront the problem of the widespread failure to provide an adequate education to underprivileged minorities such as the black children who brought this lawsuit" (p. 992).

Literacy

The significant impairment in reading and writing skills manifested by many speakers of social dialects, is a major concern to contemporary educators and habilitationists. As Wolfram, et al. (1979) have noted:

> Many educators have become increasingly alarmed at the literacy situation in American schools today. As the need for reading skills increases, so does our awareness that large numbers of people in our society do not possess adequate literacy skills. *Among the many people with significant reading problems are those who do not speak what has been labeled "standard English." Reading problems seem to be more common among nonstandard English speakers than among their standard English speaking counterparts* . . . (p. 1) italics added

Similarly, writing problems have been noted in social dialect speakers (Wolfram & Fasold, 1979). Substandard writing skills are related to a variety of factors, but it is clear that spoken dialect plays a significant role in nonstandard writing patterns.

The literacy problem — the educational retardation — of minority poor, and especially black children is still present, and our educational institutions have not succeeded in providing an adequate educational environment for them. The Ann Arbor decision in 1980 gives additional support to the need for an effective education — in this case, reading abilities at appropriate grade levels.

Educators have long considered deprivation of experiences and poor home stimulation or motivation as being the paramount causes of educational retardation. We submit that it is time to examine carefully the issues of (1) linguistic conflict and (2) deviation from the majority's culture and value system.

Social dialects, such as Black English, are rule-governed dialectal systems as standard English is a rule-governed system. Yet, it is the standard dialect rules that are taught exclusively to all children without regard for the rules of their home dialect. It is the conflict or interference among the rules that in part at least, cause the problems in literacy. The root cause of the educational retardation is not inappropriate home stimulation or motivation, as so many people apparently believe. If this were so, poor black children would come from home environments that are significantly deficient in educational stimulation — as compared to poor children from other ethnic or racial homes. This is patently not so. The only logical reason for this deficiency is the significant difference in linguistic rules, as was previously stated.

We believe, therefore, that a bidialectal and a bicultural teaching program initiated in the preschool years before reading and writing skills are taught, will help children process information more effectively. If we are to provide an adequate education for the minority poor, and especially black children, we must consider other alternatives to the current unidialectal and unicultural language arts teaching strategies.

Employment

In addition to the relationship between oral dialect and reading/writing skills, the dialect speaker may experience a social rejection by members of the middle-class; in particular, this rejection is manifested in the job market where certain kinds of employment opportunities have been severely limited for such speakers.*

One example of such discrimination was reported in the June 24, 1979 edition of *Sunday Magazine,* a supplement to the *Atlanta Journal and Constitution newspapers.* A reporter, Lee May, had applied for positions listed in the employment section of the newspaper; in each case he was rejected when he spoke in Black English as an applicant for

---

*Recent statistics point out that the unemployment among blacks is particularly high.

the position; in each case he was asked to interview when re-applying for the same position using standard English. Similar examples exist relevant to the negative impact that social dialect has upon listeners. In point of fact, many middle-class listeners are prejudicial toward such speech patterns. Such speakers frequently are assumed to be dumb* and/or inferior people.

The concern about such negative stereotypes and the harmful impact of such perceptions was indicated by the major conference sponsored by the Southern Regional Education Board (SREB) in 1979. Invited to this two and one-half day meeting were faculty and administrators of colleges with significant black populations. There were consultants in reading, writing, and this author was the specialist in oral language. The theme of the conference pertained to this negative stereotype and the employability problems of black graduates from these colleges. The concern at the conference was that students who speak or write in Black English were not learning to speak or write in standard English.

Generally, it may be said that many economically poor speakers retain the linguistic and paralinguistic patterns common to their culture; i.e., poor blacks continue to use Black English dialect, and poor Appalachians continue to use Mountain English dialect. And, as suggested above, such dialectal usage often penalizes the user in the middle-class "market-place" where standard English is assumed to be the only proper English dialect.

Social Dialect

Our understanding of dialectal differences in this country has been limited generally to regional or geographical variants of standard English such as General American dialect, or Southern dialect, etc. It is only recently that the propriety of social dialects has been examined with any sustained regularity. The works of sociolinguists such as Labov (1966, 1968), Stewart (1967, 1968), Wolfram (1969, 1975), Baratz (1969), Dillard (1972) and others have detailed the linguistic regularities of not only Black English but also the mountain speech of Appalachia and have made explicit the need for appli-

---

*This pejorative term is deliberately used, because it is believed by the author, that such impressions are, in fact, frequently generated. Although there may have been some rejections based upon race, other rejections would probably be related to the negative stereotype.

cation of these regularities. The major conception emerging from this research is that these varieties of English Black and Mountain) are complete linguistic systems in their own right, with specific rules of grammar, phonology, and lexicon, and differ basically in the fact that they are less prestigious forms of standard English.

The application of this linguistic research, however, has been difficult. In their interactions with children possessing social dialects, educators and clinicians have few options open to them, and these choices entail drastically different teaching or treating strategies. There are three feasible options available when considering a practical application of linguistic data: (1) use only standard English in the classroom or therapy room and consequently eradicate any dialectal differences; that is, reject the dialect by indicating that it is incorrect to speak in that dialect; (2) accept the dialect in the classroom without teaching its standard English equivalent; or (3) utilize a bidialectal approach which teaches both the dialect and standard English; that is, the student is taught to "switch" dialects (to manifest diglossic behavior) according to the demands of the speaking situation. In previous publications, we have contended that the theoretical framework of bidialectalism provides the best alternative (Adler, 1971 a,b,c, 1973, 1976, 1978, 1979, 1981). Proponents of compensatory or "enrichment" education have utilized the first technique (i.e., teaching only through standard English) with apparently little success. Programs designed around the second concept handicap individuals by not teaching them effectively the prestigious "standard" dialect, which is the predominant medium of higher education, business, and government. The bidialectal approach teaches speakers to compare and contrast their own dialect with standard English. Jaggar and Cullinan (1974) suggest that the native dialect should be respected and maintained but that the goal of the language programs is to help those who speak a non-standard dialect to add another dialect, i.e., standard English, to their repertoire.

LANGUAGE TEACHING

It may be said that most conventional language arts teaching strategies, which are usually eradicationist, or non-interventionist, are not sufficiently effective with poor children. Too many of these children are not learning to be speakers of standard English. Instead, they retain those linguistic and paralinguistic patterns common to their culture; i.e., poor blacks continue to use Black English dialect, and poor Appalachians continue to use Mountain English dialect. And, as previously emphasized, this affects their acquisition of standard reading and writing skills.

There has been very little research that either supports or contradicts the bidialectal position. Feigenbaum (1970) constructed a program for use in high schools around the foreign language methodology of contrastive analysis. In this method, labels are given to the different languages or dialects being taught (e.g., "formal" for standard English and "informal" for the nonstandard dialect), and students are taught, through exercises and pattern drills, to differentiate between the two. Leaverton (1969) and his associates in Chicago used the same methodology to design a first grade reading program for black children. This program used dialect readers to explain the differences between "everyday" and "school" talk. Somerville (1975) has noted that this program has had some success.

Research is also sparse in teaching standard English as a second dialect before reading instruction begins. Rystrom conducted two experiments with first grade groups, one in California (1968) and the other in Georgia (1970). Experimental groups of black children received training in standard English twenty minutes a day for eight weeks in the California study, and for six months in the Georgia study. Pre- and post-testing with the Gates Word Reading Test and sections of the Standard Achievement Test revealed no significant difference for the experimental and control groups. However, Somerville (1975) noted that both studies were initiated well into the school year and were conducted concurrently with reading instruction. Also, Rystrom (1970) pointed out that the simultaneous presentation of dialect training and reading instruction seemed to have been confusing to the children. Clayton's (1974) three month study of kindergarten through third grade children from Morgan County, Tennessee, was the first program to utilize the bidialectal approach successfully with rural Appalachian children.

DEVELOPING A BIDIALECTAL PROGRAM

During our tenure as consultant to the Knox County, Tennessee, Head Start Programs, we were able to initiate a two year program comparing conventional unidialectal language teaching to bidialectal language teaching. Children in three classes were used as the experimental group, and children in three other classes were used as the control group during the first year, and seven classes for both experimental and control groups were used in the second year.* The following dynamics were utilized in the bidialectal program.

Dialectal Patterns

An important prerequisite before the actual teaching program began was the determination of exactly what specific items of dialect were encountered in the primarily white population in this Appalachian area. The work of other authors in northern cities and West Virginia (Labov, 1966, Wolfram, 1969, 1975) was used as a reference guide for the collection of the speech samples. Several methods were used to collect the samples: (1) The primary method used was spontaneous transcription while a given child was in the classroom, in therapy sessions, or in small play groups; (2) another method involved analysis of certain test response items differing from standard English; (3) also, remote telemetry recordings were used that allowed taping of children in therapy or at play in our day care center program (The Pediatric Language Laboratory). An effort was made to take samples from each child in both the school environment and the playground situation.

Once the samples were taken, they were analyzed by noting the similarities and differences in grammatical, lexical, and phonological output between the language of the children and the standard English spoken in the geographic area. Standard English was operationally defined as the socially prestigious language patterns accepted and used by middle-class speakers in this East Tennessee region, particularly the school teachers in this area. Members of the child's cultural community were then questioned to ascertain if the dialectal features were still prominent in the area. A "dialectal difference" then was defined as a phonological, grammatical, and/or lexical feature manifested by the child which was in current use in

---

*All subjects were members of the lower social classes, as dictated by Head Start policies; most were white, but some were black; they ranged in age from 3.0 to 6.0 years. The information being presented is also relevant to early elementary classrooms in which a similar study was done, and similar results generated.

the child's cultural community, and which also differed from the standard English spoken in the geographic area.

Teaching Strategy

In general, the teaching strategy was designed around two broad ideas, as suggested by Labov (1973) and Wolfram (1970). Labov notes the advantages in teaching the general items of the different dialects. He states that some non-standard forms are special cases that affect only one or two words of the language; but many are instances of general rules that operate in the nonstandard vernacular in a regular way and can affect the form of every sentence. Labov believes, therefore, that the more general rules should be introduced first in a teaching program. Wolfram makes the additional observation that it is important to teach the standard English form of socially stigmatized dialectal variants first in any program. The suggestions of Labov and Wolfram were incorporated into the teaching program.

Teacher In-Service Programs

The acceptance by the teachers of Mountain English and Black English as distinct and valid linguistic systems proved to be the most difficult aspect of this bidialectal program. To promote an understanding of this concept, several in-service sessions were conducted which attempted to explain previous research and clarify issues involved in the programs. These teachers were visited at least once a week to eliminate problems, to check on the progress made by the children, and to supply the teachers with new lesson plans. Control and experimental teachers were paired as to their educational background and work experience.

The Contrastive Analysis Approach: Everyday vs School Talk

The specific lesson plans for this program were centered around the contrastive analysis approach. Johnson (1971) describes the five steps inherent in the use of this approach. A child must (1) recognize that there is a difference between his language and the language he is learning, (2) hear the target language sound or grammatical pattern, (3) discriminate between his language and the target language at the conflict points, (4) reproduce the target language feature and (5) practice the target language feature in oral drills. The labels of "school"-talk and "everyday"-talk were used to differentiate between standard English and the child's dialect.

Special situations were created in order to facilitate the discrimination between "everyday" and "school" talk. Hand puppets were used in the early stages of the program, i.e., an "everyday" puppet and a "school" puppet. Later, pictures which represented a school or everyday environment were presented with the child identifying various speech-language patterns as appropriate to each. Finally, role-playing was instituted; e.g., the child could assume the role of mother, father, teacher or businessman. Varied contexts made the material presented more entertaining for the children and sustained their attention for longer periods of time.

The program was divided into two interrelated phases:

Phase I consisted of a fifteen minute formal language instruction period in which the teacher compared and contrasted the features of the target language with standard English, using the lesson plans described above. Each class received instruction once a day, Monday through Friday (see the Appendix for examples).

Phase II consisted of reinforcement of the differences between school — and every — day — talk by the teacher or her aide at various times throughout the day. Using informal situations such as recess or lunch, this method consisted of the teacher verbally rewarding the children for their appropriate use of school and everyday talk patterns.

Teacher Response

Teacher comments suggested that bidialectal teaching may be more effective than the more conventional unidialectal approach as in the eradicationist strategy. Not only did the children tend to use more standard English sentences, but they also seemed to communicate more, as one teacher said "to open up more in the classroom."

Initially, there was a good deal of teacher resistance to the program; one teacher, in fact, made it clear that she was cooperating only because she was told to do so. But our in-service programs and informal meetings with the teaching staff, as well as the involvement and cooperation of a Head-Start speech-language clinician, soon generated a positive relationship. The feed back from the teachers was generally positive and supportive of the program. It is clear that such cooperation is a necessity, if the program is to succeed, but that this cooperation is not easily obtained.

POLITICAL & SOCIAL IMPLICATION

There are political and social reasons why the implementation of a bidialectal teaching program is difficult to initiate. Politically, school administrators — as well as teachers and speech clinicians — are hesitant to implement such a program because of public condemnation. As long as the lay public believes that social dialects are substandard, they will have much difficulty accepting the teaching of this information in the classroom. Socially, people have been conditioned to believe that social dialect patterns are incorrect and substandard and require remediation. This belief makes it difficult for many middle-class parents to comprehend why we want to teach these English patterns.

Communication specialists must be aware that such dialects are not substandard and that their effective utilization will allow for more effective learning of standard English. As the discipline best prepared to accept the responsibility for teaching bidialectalism (Adler, 1971a), it is incumbent upon speech-language pathologists to teach these concepts to teachers and to point out that the most common approaches to social dialects, the eradication and nonintervention approaches, have not been successful. Therefore, it is time to try something else. In their places, we recommend the bidialectal approach (Adler & Tims, 1980).

THE IMPLICATIONS OF PROFICIENCY TEST SCORES TO BIDIALECTAL TEACHING

Support for bidialectal teaching is fueled by scores on proficiency (or competency) tests. These scores are related to the children's social class membership. That is, economically poor children score poorer on these tests than do their middle-class counterparts.

There are a number of factors that contribute to these low scores, but dialect interference and conflict and ensuing communication difficulties play a significant role. The effective teaching of standard (local) English should assume a very important role, and speech-language clinicians should teach the appropriate bidialectal concepts to the teachers.

CONCLUSION

Many speech-language clinicians, as well as educators and other professional workers, treat social dialects by attempting to eradicate them or by accepting them, i.e., the non-intervention approach. Both of these philosophies have proven, in general, to be ineffective: (1) the dialectal patterns are not being eradicated; standard English is not being used by many or most of the minority poor students in our schools; (2) the acceptance of dialectal patterns is potentially deleterious to educational acquisition or literacy, and to employment in certain occupations. Hence, both the non-intervention philosophy and the eradicationist approach are considered to be unacceptable.

The funtion of the clinician is to teach these concepts of bidialectalism to educators and to apply them in the therapy room.

Appendix

A SAMPLE OF THE BIDIALECTAL LESSON PLANS USED IN THE KNOX COUNTY HEAD-START PROGRAM*

Lesson Plan A

Purpose: The purpose of this lesson plan is to contrast phonological, grammatical and lexical features of standard and nonstandard English.

Materials: These allow you to present a visual presentation of the vocabulary to be taught.

Level P Peabody Vocabulary cards
      F - 22 & F - 35
      T - 16
      H - 1 & H - 18

*We wish to acknowledge the help of Diane File in the development of these lesson plans.

Vocabulary to be Contrasted:

Everyday Talk	School Talk
Tater	Potatoe
Clum	Climbed
Pert'n Near	Almost

Sentences to be Contrasted:

1. Ilike to eat *tater* chips.   vs.   Ilike to eat *potatoe* chips.
   Momma fixed a baked *tater.*   vs.   Momma fixed a baked *potatoe.*
2. I *clum* the jungle gym (monkey bars).   vs.   I *climbed* the jungle gym (monkey bars).
3. It's purt'n near time for my bath (Sesame Street, etc.)   vs.   It's *almost* time for my bath. (Sesame Street, etc.)

Activities Using Previously Learned Vocabulary:

1. Take the children for a walk on the playground. Talk about the everyday things you see — birds, trees, grass, etc. Have each child bring back to class an everyday thing and tell something about it during group time.
2. Teach the children new vocabulary using school tools, e.g. chalk, eraser, blackboard. Place several items in a row, blindfold a child and remove an item. Take the blindfold off the child and have him name the missing object.
3. Do the same, using both school and everyday objects. Have the child identify what's missing and tell whether it's an everyday or school item.

Lesson Plan B

Purpose: The purpose of this lesson plan is to contrast grammatical, phonological and lexical items off standard and nonstandard English.

Materials: These allow you to present a visual representation of the vocabulary to be taught. P-8; H-32; A-39; C-7; P-25; Level P Peabody Vocabulary Cards.

Vocabulary to be Contrasted:

Everyday Talk	School Talk	
Bresh	Brush	(P-8 & H-32)
Whar	Where	(C-7)
Reckon	Believe	(P-25)
Be	Is	(A-39)

Sentences to be Contrasted:

1. I can *bresh* my hair, clothes, etc.   vs.   I can *brush* my hair, clothes, etc.
2. This one *be* a butterfly.   vs.   This one *is* a butterfly.
3. *Whar* are my jeans?   vs.   *Where* are my jeans?
4. I *reckon* she is crying.   vs.   I *believe* she is crying.

Activities Using Previously Learned Vocabulary:

1. Cut a cardboard box to represent a TV screen. Let the children take turns playing weatherman. Have them describe the weather (may need to prompt to tell about the sky, what kind of clothes to wear today, etc.). Teacher will encourage a series of sentences using everyday and school talk.

2. Plan a pretend picnic. Let the children select pictures of everyday things to put in the picnic basket. Later, have the children draw a picture about the picnic.

3. Organize a store; stock it with various items. Give each child ten "pennies". Each item in the store will cost from 1 to 10 cents. The child must ask for an item using everyday or school talk. The teacher tells the child the price of the item and the child pays the appropriate amount.

Lesson Plan C

Purpose: The purpose of this lesson plan is to contrast prosodic features of standard and nonstandard English.

The prosodic features — rhythm, melody, rate and stress (force) — make language more expressive. Syllables and words can be compared to an accordion — they can be stretched out or compressed. In speech, some utterances are "drawn out" to express contentment, weariness, reverence, awe or deep grief. Utterances may also be compressed to express an extreme emotional state — fear, rage or excitement.

Non-standard English may be characterized by slow, quiet timing in speech with a pause between syllables and words. In standard English, these pauses may create an uncomfortable feeling in the listener and/or speaker.

To help the children become more aware of these contrasts, demonstrate and contrast fast and slow rhythms through clapping, beating drums, tapping marching, walking, etc. Talk about the differences as you demonstrate the rhythms. Perhaps the teacher could demonstrate one form (e.g., fast) and her aide, the other (e.g., slow). Demonstrate them, then have the children repeat them. Have the children do them with you.

Vocabulary To Be Contrasted:

	Everyday Talk		School Talk
1.	Counting: o-n-e-; t-wo; th-r-ee; etc.	vs.	one; two; three
2.	Sa- a - a - ad	vs.	Sad
3.	N - o - o - o	vs.	No

Activities Using previously Learned Vocabulary:

1. Ask a child to count the other children in the circle using everyday (school) talk. Ask the remaining children whether he(she) used everyday (school) talk. One day, have all the children count using everyday talk. The next day, have them count using school talk.

2. As the children go from group time to another activity, explain to them that they have a choice between two activities. To get to the next activity, they must ask the teacher (aide), "May I go to the _____?" If they do not ask "May I", the teacher (aide) will respond using the everyday (school) form "No (n-o-o-o) you cannot go to the _____."
   Once in the playground, line the children up to play "May I." The teacher (aide) can be "IT." The children must ask "May I take two small steps?" etc. If children say "May I," they are allowed to take the steps, etc. If not, the reply is "No (N-o-o-o) you may not take _____." First child to reach "IT" becomes the new "IT."

3. Select a child from the group and ask him(her to put on a "Happy Face." Ask the other children, "Is _____ sad (sa-a-ad)?"

Have them reply using everyday (school) talk, "No (n-o-o-o), _____ isn't sad (sa-a-ad)."

Dress the children up. Explain that they are going to town to grocery shop. The teacher (aide) may be the clerk. The children go into the store and ask, "Do you have any ____ for sale," the clerk will reply, "No (n-o-o-o), I don't have any ____ for sale." Let the children take turns being the clerk, explaining to them they must use the everyday (school) talk way to say "No."

REFERENCES

Adler, S. Dialectal Differences: Professional and Clinical Implications. *Journal of Speech and Hearing Disorders,* 1971a, *36,* 9-100.

. Pluralism, Relevance, and Language Intervention. *ASHA,* 1971b, *36* 719-725.

. A Sociolinguistic Approach to Functional Mental Retardation. *Exceptional Children,* 1971c, *38,* 336-337.

. Social Class Bases of Language: A Reexamination of Socioeconomic, Sociopsychological, and Sociolinguistic Factors. *ASHA,* 1973, *38,* 3-9.

. A Language Intervention Program for Culturally Different Children. *Communicative Disorders: An Audio Journal for Continuing Education,* New York, NY: Grune and Stratton, Inc., 1976.

. Language Intervention and the Culturally Different Child. *School Psychology Digest,* 1978, *7,* 16-26.

. *Poverty Children and Their Language: Implications for Teaching and Treating Strategies,* New York, NY: Grune & Stratton, Inc. 1979.

. Testing: Considerations in Cultural Differences. *Seminars in Speech, Language and Hearing,* 1981, *2,* 77-90.

Adler, S., & Tims, I. A. W. The Pediatric Language Specialist: An Innovative Approach to Early Language Intervention and the Role of the Speech-Language Clinician. In N. J. Lass (Ed.), *SPEECH AND LANGUAGE: Advances in Basic Research & Practice.* New York, NY: Academic Press, Inc., 1980.

Baratz, J. Teaching Reading in an Urban Negro School System. In J. Baratz & R. Shuy (Ed.s), *Teaching Black Children to Read.* Washington, DC: Center for Applied Linguistics, 1969.

Bountress, N. G. The Ann Arbor Decision: Implications for the Speech-Language Pathologists. *ASHA,* 1980, *22,* 543-544.

Clayton, K. Evaluation of the Effectiveness of a Short-term Program Employing A Bidialectal Method of Teaching Language to White American Children. Unpublished Master's Thesis, Knoxville: University of Tennessee, 1974.

Dillard, J. L. *Black English: Its History and Usage in the United States, New York:* Random House, 1972.

Feigenbaum, I. The Use of Nonstandard English in Teaching Standard: Contrast and Comparison. In R. Fasold & R. Shuy (Eds.), *Teaching Standard English in the Inner City.* Washington, DC: Center for Applied Linguistics, 1970.

Jaggar, A. M., & Cullinan, B. E. Teaching Standard English to Achieve Bidialectalism: Problems with Current Practices. *Florida FL Reporter,* 1974, Spring & Fall, 63-70.

Johnson, K. R. Should Black Children Learn Standard English? In M. Imhoof (Ed.), Viewpoints, *Bulletin of the School of Education,* Indiana University, 1971, *47,* 83-101.

Labov, W. *The Social Stratification of English in New York City.* Washington, DC: Center for Applied Linguistics, 1966.

Labov, W., Cohen, P., Robins, C. & Lewis, J. *A Study of the Non-Standard English of Negro and Puerto Rican Speakers in New York City.* USOE Final Report, Research Project No. 3288, 1968.

Labor, W., & Cohen, P. Some Suggestions for Teaching Standard English to Speakers of Nonstandard and Urban Dialects. In J. DeStefano (Ed.), *Language, Society, and Education: A Profile of Black English.* Worthington, OH: Wadsworth Publishing Co., 1973.

Leaverton, L., Davis, O., & Gladney, M. *The Psycholinguistics Reading Series: A Bidialectal Approach.* Chicago: Board of Education, 1969.

May, L. Black English. In Atlanta Journal & Constitution newspaper, *Sunday Magazine,* June 24, 1979.

Rystrom, R. C. Dialect Training and Reading: A Further Look. *Reading Research Quarterly,* 1970, *40,* 581-599.

Somerville, M. Dialect and Reading: A Review of Alternative Solutions. *Review of Educational Research,* 1975, 45:2, 247-262. Chicago: Board of Education.

Stewart, W. A. Continuity and Change in American Negro Dialects. *Florida FL Reporter, 1968, 6,* 14-16, 18, 304.

The Ann Arbor Decision, Memorandum, Opinion & Order, & The Education Plan. Arlington, VA: Center for Applied Linguistics, 1979.

Whiteman, M. F. (Ed.) *Reactions to Ann Arbor: Vernacular Black English & Education, Introduction.* Arlington, VA: Center for Applied Linguistics, 1980.

Wolfram, W. *A Sociolinguistic Description of Detroit Negro Speech.* Washington, D.C.: Center for Applied Linguistics, 1969.

　　Sociolinguistic Implications for Educational Sequencing. In R. Fasold and R. Shuy (Eds.), *Teaching Standard English in the Inner City.* Washington, D.C.: Center for Applied Linguistics, 1970.

Wolfram, W, & Christian, D. *Sociolinguistic Variables in Appalachian Dialects.* Arlington, VA: Center for Applied Linguistics, 1975.

Wolfram , W., & Fasold, R. Social Dialects and Education. In J.B. Pride (Ed.), *Sociolinguistic Aspects of Language Learning & Teaching (section 4).* Oxford, England: Oxford University Press, 1979.

Wolfram, W., Potter, L., Yanofsky, N., & Shuy R. *Reading & Dialect Differences.* Arlington, VA: Center for Applied Linguistics, 1979.

Chapter III

THE RELATIONSHIP OF ENGLISH COMPOSITION GRADES TO ORAL (SOCIAL) DIALECT:

An Analysis of Dialectal and Non-Dialectal Writing Errors

KENDALL RUSSELL BERGIN

INTRODUCTION

Dialect Diversity and Education

AS the principal means used for the transmission of information, language plays a significant role in the educational process. The importance of this role is most pointedly realized in individuals who use a variety of American English different from that adopted as the standard by the majority of American English speakers. Because the educational process necessitates verbal and written use of the accepted standard, students who have previously mastered and implemented a different variety of American English for oral communication may experience limited academic success.

The purpose of the college English composition course is to develop the students' ability to use the written form of American English in communication. Although many varieties of American

29

English are spoken, the variety used in the educational classroom is that adopted by the majority of American English speakers. This variety is commonly referred to as standard English. Two other varieties of American English are commonly spoken by members of the speech community, Black English (Ebonics) and Appalachian or Mountain English. These two varieties are referred to as non-standard English or oral (social) dialects because: (1) they differ from the standard English variety, (2) they are spoken by members of similar sociocultural and/or sociolinguistic backgrounds* and (3) they are not recognized by the "establishment" as a means of transmitting information other than through social dialogue. These non-standard English dialects as well as the standard English pattern have been demonstrated to be fully formed linguistic systems (Wolfram and Whiteman, 1971; Labov, 1970).

Dialect and English Composition

The relationship of oral (social) dialect usage to writing errors and success in the English composition course remains to be thoroughly explored. The purpose of this study was to therefore define and describe those relationships as they exist among three sociolinguistically different groups of students.

Students who speak a non-standard variety of English enter the classroom with a language system that can rarely be applied in composition. Because the academic community accepts and adopts as its standard the standard English language system, the social dialect speaker is more likely to encounter writing difficulties and thus to achieve less academic success. This is confirmed in part from the difficulties that non-standard English speakers have been observed to have with the written language form (Shaughnessy, 1977) and in part by observations of student writing errors made by English composition instructors (Wolfram & Whiteman, 1971).

Classroom Performance Differences

Differences in educational performance between non-standard and standard English speakers are often noted in the classroom (Shaughnessy, 1977). Wolfram and Fasold (1979) maintain that

---

*The term socio-cultural refers to the familial heritage, values, patterns of belief and environmental experiences associated with an individual.

The term socio-linguistic refers to the establishment and use of language by individuals within their social environment.

when the value system of the educational system matches that sector of society from which the children come and when the notion of what is correct in speech matches that acquired at home, the process of education is served well. However, Wolfram and Fasold (1979) additionally maintain that a mismatch between the non-standard dialect users values and language system with that of the educational system, overwhelms the individual who has communicated effectively with his/her nonstandard patterns in the home and community.

Shaughnessy (1977) observed that toward the end of the sixties, many four-year colleges were admitting students who were not ready to undertake the traditional academic coursework. More specifically, Shaughnessy noted that:

> when the City University of New York adopted an admissions policy that guaranteed to every city resident a place in one of its eighteen tuition-free colleges . . . a wider range of students than any college had probably ever admitted or thought of admitting to its campus — academic winners and losers from the best and worst high schools in the country, the children of the lettered and illiterate, the blue collared, and the unemployed — reflected the city's intense, troubled version of America.

Similar changes were occurring in educational institutions across America bringing not only nontraditional students into the classroom but nonstandard dialects as well.

The difficulties that nonstandard dialect speakers experience in the academic environments of colleges and universities have been scarcely explored. Wolfram and Whiteman (1971) maintain that many of the classroom problems faced by these students stem from the language difficulties which non-standard English speaking students have in learning to read and write standard English. With particular regard to writing skills, the surface feature of oral (social) dialects may interfere with written productions of standard English forms (Epes, *et al.*, 1978; Wolfram and Whiteman, 1971).

STATEMENT OF THE PROBLEM

Success in English composition courses at the college/university level depends upon a student's ability to express concepts, ideas, and observations in writing through the use of standard English. The students who speak a dialect other than standard English, i.e., nonstandard English, might therefore be at a disadvantage in this academic situation unless they have mastered two sets of language rules, those governing their non-standard English system and those governing the standard English system.

The role oral (social) dialect usage assumes in the English composition course remains to be systematically studied. Although some research has been conducted to demonstrate that speakers of non-standard dialect experience difficulty with writing standard English (Wolfram and Whiteman, 1971), little is known about the relationship concerning the amount of oral (social) dialect usage, number of written errors, and success or failure in the college English composition course.

PURPOSE

The purposes of this study were: (1) the investigation of oral (social) dialect usage among three socio-culturally and socio-linguistically defined groups of college students (lower-middle and upper and lower-lower class rural and urban blacks; lower-middle and upper and lower-lower class rural Applachian whites; upper-middle class rural and urban whites*) enrolled in freshman English composition, (2) the investigation of the relationship among oral (social) dialect usage and number of writing errors and (3) the investigation of the relationship between oral (social) dialect usage and overall performance in the freshman English composition course as reflected in the final grades achieved by students in the three groups.

HYPOTHESES

The following hypotheses were put to appropriate statistical tests:

1. A significant difference was expected to be found in the amount of oral (social) dialect usage among the three groups. The upper-middle class rural and urban white group was expected to be significantly different from the other two groups.

2. A significant positive correlation was expected to be revealed

---

*Members of this group were assumed to be most closely associated with standard English usage. They therefore served as a control for comparisons made in this study.

between oral (social) dialect usage and number of writing errors. Students who exhibited more oral (social) dialect usage were expected to make more writing errors.

3. A significant positive correlation was expected to be revealed between oral (social) dialect usage and course performance as measured by final grades in freshman English composition. Students who exhibited more oral (social) dialect usage were expected to make poorer grades than those who exhibited little oral (social) dialect usage.

SUBJECTS

Subjects were selected from students enrolled in English 1010, Freshman English Composition during the 1982 academic year at The University of Tennessee, Knoxville. A total of 35 subjects were selected from approximately 350 students enrolled in 16 sections of English 1010.

An initial pool of subject candidates was obtained through student consent. Each student enrolled in English 1010 responded to a *Consent to Participate* form. Those students giving their consent to participate as subjects in this study became members of the initial population pool.

Subject candidates in the initial population pool responded to a *Student Information Sheet* (SIS). The purpose of the *SIS* was to identify three subgroups of subject candidates. These three subgroups are defined below:

Group I: Lower-middle, upper-lower and lower-lower class rural and urban blacks

1. Origin
   a. Geographical region: United States
   b. Community: Farm or open country; town or city of less than 10,000 population and/or indication of rural community on *SIS*; city or town with a population of 10,000 or more and/or indication of urban community on *SIS*.
2. Social class
   a. Mother's or guardian's education level: Lower-middle class 10-12 years; upper-lower class 6-9 years; lower-lower class 0-5 years.

Group II: Lower-middle, upper-lower and lower-lower class rural Appalachian whites
1. Origin
    a. Geographical region: Southern Appalachia (West Virginia, Eastern Kentucky, East Tennessee, Northeast Georgia, Northwest South Carolina, Western North Carolina, Western Virginia, and Northeast Alabama; Wolfram, 1976).
    b. Community: Farm or open country; town or city of less than 10,000 population and/or indication of rural community on *SIS*.
2. Social class
    a. Mother's or guardian's education level: Lower-middle class 10-12 years; upper-lower class 6-9 years; lower-lower class 0-5 years.

Group III: Upper-middle class rural and urban whites
1. Origin
    a. Geographical region: United States
    b. Community: Rural-farm or open country; town or city of less than 10,000 population and/or indication of rural community on *SIS* or urban-city or town with a population of 10,000 or more and/or indication of urban community on *SIS*.
2. Social class
    a. Mother's or guardian's education level: Upper-middle class 13 years and over (college).

The previously stated criteria used to define the three subject groups were imposed to obtain more homogeneous subject samples. Socio-linguistic and socio-cultural differences have been demonstrated to exist among individuals of various racial/ethnic, geographical, community and social class backgrounds (Adler, 1979; Anastasiow and Hanes, 1976; Helton, 1974; Williams, 1970; Shuy, 1967).* In addition to these criteria, subjects manifested no gross auditory, visual or motor handicaps as determined from information obtained on the *SIS*.

---

*Based on the research of Helton (1974) and proposed system of Adler (1979) maternal education level was the criterion for social class distinction.

A total of thirty-five students participated in this study. The lower-middle class black group had nine students. The lower-middle and lower class rural Appalachian white group had ten students and the upper-middle class (UMC) white group had sixteen students. The number of subjects in each group by social class distinction can be found in Table 3-I.*

Table 3-I

SOCIAL CLASS DISTINCTIONS BASED ON MATERNAL EDUCATION
LEVEL OF SUBJECT PARTICIPANTS BY GROUP

| Group | | *Social Class* | | | |
		Upper-Middle (13yrs. & over)	Lower-Middle (10-12 yrs.)	Upper-Lower (6-9 yrs.)	Lower-Lower (0-5 yrs.)
Group	I		6	2	1
Group	II		5	4	1
Group	III	16			

*Social class distinctions were used for grouping of subjects. Within group distinctions were not further utilized due to the smallness of each group.

DATA COLLECTION

Oral Dialect

The *Oral Dialect Rating Scale* was created to determine oral (social) dialect usage. The purpose of this scale was to identify the amount of oral (social) nonstandard dialect utilized by a speaker. This scale differentiated dialectal usage via an ordinal classification system. The values assigned to this scale are defined below:

1. Standard English is predominately used for communication with occasional or some difference(s) noted.
2. A dialect other than standard English is moderately used for communication in conjunction with standard English patterns.
3. A dialect other than standard English is predominately used for communication. (Pitch, rhythm, intonation patterns and/or body movements which differ from those commonly used by standard English speakers are included in this rating.)

Administration of this scale required that the evaluator: (1) be able to recognize and differentiate standard English dialect usage from other dialectal patterns such as Black English and Appalachian speech and (2) have contact with the verbal patterns of the individual being rated. Six instructors of English 1010 were assumed to meet both of these requirements and administered this scale to subjects in their section following individual conferences approximately four weeks after the course began and following classroom contact with the oral patterns of students.

Inter-judge reliability was determined from instructor ratings of a tape recorded speech sample obtained from six subjects (two from each group). The recorded sample contained 30-second response to the question "What do you have to do to write a paper for your English 1010 Course?" A percent agreement of 72.2% was obtained for the six English 1010 instructors participating in this study.

Intra-judge reliability was determined from instructor ratings of the tape recorded sample described above. These ratings were made after the first four weeks of the quarter and again one week prior to the end of the quarter. The eight samples were reordered prior to the second rating to control for possible practice effects. A percent agreement of 70% was obtained from these ratings.

One factor which may have influenced instructor ratings of oral dialect is that of familiarity with the dialect. Since the instructors have lived and taught in the Appalachian region, Appalachian English may not be as readily distinguishable from standard English mildly characterized by some of the pronunciation differences, e.g. use of dipthongs, also observed in Appalachian English. In addition, all instructors who participated were white and therefore Black English usage may have been more readily identifiable due to less personal contact with Black English patterns. These considerations are supported in part from oral reports of instructors who indicated that the dialect rating task was "hard" and that some students were easier to rate than others.

It should also be noted that only moderate percentages of agreement were obtained for inter-judge and inter-judge reliability measures. This implies that each judge was employing a somewhat different criterion for dialect usage when making the ratings. A training task for judges prior to data collection would have possibly served to eliminate some of the observed variability in ratings.

Writing Errors

Writing errors from two categories of error, grammar and spelling, were determined from two in-class papers submitted by each subject in fulfillment of English 1010 requirements. These papers were evaluated by the English 1010 instructors in accordance with the guidelines of *The Freshman English Program at The University of Tennessee.* Errors were marked according to the *Harbrace* (1977) system. The total number of errors made in grammar and spelling were calculated for each subject from the first 200 words of each paper. The instructor initially marked errors and this total was calculated for each subject. The examiner re-evaluated the writing errors of five papers according to the *Harbrace* system for determination of interjudge reliability. A Pearson product moment correlation coefficient of .97 was obtained.

Grade

The final grade was obtained for each subject from instructor grade sheets. These grades were determined by the English 1010 instructors according to the student's overall performance in the course. The final grade reflects: (1) the ability to interpret what has been read and to write coherently and comfortably about it, (2) knowledge of the fundamental principles of English grammar, (3) the ability to make corrections made on class assignments and other work required and (4) the degree of competence achieved and sustained by the student (Freshman English Program Handbook 1980-81). A final grade of A, B, C, or NC was determined for each subject.

RESULTS AND DISCUSSION

The purposes of this study were: (1) to investigate the oral dialect usage among three socio-culturally and socio-linguistically defined groups of freshman English 1010 (Written Composition) students, (2) to investigate the relationship between oral dialect usage and number of writing errors made by those students and (3) to investigate the relationship between oral dialect usage and success in the freshman English composition course as reflected by the final grade achieved by students in the three groups. Data for students participating in the study were obtained in cooperation with the Department of English at The University of Tennessee, Knoxville during Winter Quarter, 1982. Table 3-II contains a summary of raw data for each student by group.

Oral Dialect Usage of Subject Groups

The oral dialect rating data (Table 3-III) indicate that only the lower-middle and lower class black group was significantly different in dialect usage from the other two groups, lower-middle and lower class Appalachian whites and upper-middle class (UMC) whites. The dialect usage of Apalachian whites and UMC whites was not significantly different. Three possible explanations should be considered: 1) the criteria used to differentiate among groups of non-standard English speakers were not adequate, 2) the desired subject population was not available, and 3) instructors of the English composition course were able to identify Black English patterns from standard English but experienced difficulty differentiating Appalachian English from standard English.

Oral Dialect Usage and Number of English Composition Errors

There was a significant positive relationship between oral dialect usage and the number of writing errors for the subject population. This indicates that students who exhibit more non-standard oral language make more writing errors. These findings support observations made by Epes, et al. (1978) and Wolfram and Whiteman (1971), who indicated that the surface features of oral dialect might interfere with written production of standard English forms.

Further analysis of the relationship between oral dialect ratings and number of writing errors by group revealed a strong positive relationship for blacks and a very weak relationship for Appalachian whites and UMC whites. Thus, for the black subjects, an increased amount of non-standard dialect usage was associated with an increased amount of writing errors. Appalachian and UMC whites exhibited standard English or standard English with some non-standard differences noted (with the exception of one Appalachian white subject) and did not demonstrate a strong relationship between oral dialect ratings and number of writing errors. The one Appalachian white who received a "3" rating indicating non-standard English usage had the maximum observed number of writing errors, 52.

Table 3-II

DIALECT RATINGS, NUMBER OF WRITING ERRORS AND GRADE IN ENGLISH 1010 FOR SUBJECT PARTICIPANTS

Group/Subject		Dialect Rating	Data Writing Errors	Grade
	1	2	13	NC**
	2	3	.*	NC
I	3	3	.	NC
(LMC, ULC,	4	2	6	B
LLC blacks)	5	2	11	C
	6	1	22	C
	7	3	23	NC
	8	3	16	NC
	9	2	12	NC
	10	1	12	C
	11	2	29	NC
II	12	1	11	C
(LMC, ULC, LLC	13	2	15	C
Appalachian Whites)	14	1	5	B
	15	1	12	C
	16	1	8	C
	17	3	52	NC
	18	1	5	A
	19	2	4	C
	20	1	9	C
	21	1	1	B
	22	2	1	A
	23	2	10	C
	24	2	11	NC
III	25	1	13	NC
(UMC whites)	26	1	5	C
	27	2	7	C
	28	1	3	C
	29	1	6	B
	30	1	2	B
	31	1	2	B
	32	1	7	NC
	33	2	2	B
	34	2	6	B
	35	1	6	B

*Missing Data.
**Student received a grade of no credit (NC).

Table 3-III

DISTRIBUTION OF ORAL DIALECT RATINGS BY GROUP

Group		*Oral Dialect Rating* 1	2	3	Total
Group	I	1	4	4	9
Group	II	6	3	1	10
Group	III	10	6	0	16
Total		17	13	5	

Students who were identified as standard English users tended to produce fewer writing errors than students identified as non-standard English users. Approximately 70 percent of the students with a "1" (standard English) rating produced few errors whereas approximately 63 percent of the students with a "2" or "3" (non-standard English user) rating produced many errors. Shaughnessy (1977) has observed that there are writing errors which are common to all basic or developmental writing students. Further delineation of non-standard English users' writing errors indicate that some are traceable to non-standard dialect interference and that some are not (Swanson, 1975; Wolfram and Fasold, 1979). The results of this study support these observations. Students who utilized more oral non-standard English patterns made more writing errors, particularly the black students who had higher ratings of non-standard oral dialect.

Oral Dialect Usage and Course Performance

There was a significant positive relationship between oral dialect ratings and course performance as measured by final grades. Students who exhibited more non-standard English patterns performed poorer in the course (Table 3-IV).

Table 3-IV

DISTRIBUTION OF GRADES BY GROUP

Group		*Grade* A	B	C	NC
Group	I	0	1	2	6
Group	II	1	1	6	2
Group	III	1	7	5	3
Total		2	9	13	11

Further analysis of the relationship between oral dialect ratings and final grades by group revealed a strong positive relationship for blacks and Appalachian whites and a weak negative relationship for UMC whites. This indicates that oral dialect patterns of blacks and Appalachian whites were related to course performance. Oral dialect ratings of UMC whites were not related to course performance.

Students identified as standard English users tended to perform better in the course than students identified as nonstandard English users. Approximately 63 percent of the number of students who passed the course were identified as standard English users ("1" rating) whereas approximately 82 percent of the number of students who failed to pass the course were identified as non-standard English ("2" or "3" rating) users.

Overall there were seventeen students who received a "1" (standard English) rating and five who received a "3" (predominant use of non-standard English) rating. Fifteen of the students with a "1" rating passed the course with a grade of A, B, or C. All five students with a "3" rating failed to pass the course with a NC grade. Since the final grade reflects overall course performance, not just writing errors made on papers, it is apparent that predominately non-standard English speakers experience more difficulty than standard English speakers with other aspects related to course performance.

Consideration must be given to the possibility that the predominant non-standard dialect speaker's work is affected by dialect interference on reading assignments and in student-instructor conferences. The socio-cultural and socio-linguistic background of the non-standard English speaker is different from the socio-cultural and socio-linguistic standard English criteria adopted by the educational institution. This difference may affect the non-standard dialect speaker's understanding of what has been read due to lack of familiarity with the content or standard English grammatical forms. Socio-cultural and socio-linguistic differences reflected in vocabulary, grammar and body language may also affect the communication interchange between the instructor and student.

Two-thirds of the group which demonstrated higher non-standard dialect ratings, lower-middle and lower class blacks, failed to pass the course. Generally, black students had more difficulty with the course than students in the other two groups. The Appalachian white student who demonstrated predominant non-standard dialect usage also received a NC grade indicating course performance problems.

These results serve to confirm informal observations made by the English instructors who participated in this study: students who demonstrate non-standard English patterns experience more difficulty with the course and thus make poorer grades.

Implications for the Non-standard English Speaker

In the freshman English composition course, the non-standard English speaker must demonstrate written competence in standard English. The results of this study suggest that students who exhibit non-standard oral dialect tend to make more writing errors and perform more poorly in the course. This was particularly evident for the black subjects studied. Many of those students may therefore repeat the course only to experience the same difficulties because they have not mastered the oral and written standard English language systems.

Since non-standard English patterns such as Black English and Appalachian English have been identified as fully formed linguistic systems (Labov, 1970; Wolfram and Whiteman, 1971), the non-standard oral dialect user may therefore be unable to write with standard English until she/he can speak standard English.

The implications of this research clearly demonstrate the necessity of teaching non-standard speakers, particularly those with enough non-standard dialect to warrant "3" ratings, oral standard English before they are enrolled in a standard English writing course. The conflict between the non-standard and standard dialects will cause non-standard speakers to experience continued difficulty in the freshman English writing classes unless such conflict is resolved. Additional consideration should be given to the possible effect of non-standard English usage on other courses. Since non-standard English usage affects performance in the freshman English composition course, it may also affect performance in other courses.

The development of an oral communication laboratory where those non-standard English speakers desirous of learning student English have this opportunity appears to be needed at the University of Tennessee. Based on the results of this study, the contention is that non-standard English users would improve their writing skills through mastery of oral standard English as compared to the writing skills of non-standard English users not enrolled in an oral dialect laboratory.

REFERENCES

Adler, Sol. *Poverty Children and Their Language*. New York: Grune and Stratton, 1979.

Anastasiow, Nicholas J., and Michael L. Hanes. *Language Patterns of Poverty Children*. Springfield, IL: Charles C Thomas, 1976.

Epes, Mary, *et al*. "Investigating Error in the Writing of Non-traditional College Student." Paper presented at the Annual Meeting of the Modern Language Association of America (93rd, New York City, December 27-30, 1978). ERIC Document ED 168018, 1978.

Hays, William L. *Statistics for the Social Sciences*. 2nd ed. New York: Holt, Rinehart and Winston, 1973.

Helton, John Russell. "The Value of Occupation, Education, and Income In Predicting PPVT Scores of Preshcool-Aged Children; Some Comments On Criteria Commonly Utilized for Social Class Stratification." Unpublished Thesis, University of Tennessee, Knoxville, 1974.

Labov, William. "The Logic of Non-standard English." *Language and Poverty*. Ed. F. Williams. Chicago: Markham, 1970.

Shaughnessy, Mina P. *Errors and Expectations*. New York: Oxford University Press. 1977.

Shuy, Roger W. *Discovering American Dialects*. Urbana, IL: National Council of Teachers of English, 1967.

Swanson, Carol. "Linguistics and the Crisis in Writing." Paper presented at the Annual Meeting of the Linguistics Association (November 1975). ERIC Document ED 126520, 1975.

Williams, Fredrick. "Some Preliminaries and Prospects." *Language and Poverty*. Ed. Fredrick Williams. Chicago: Markham, 1970.

Wolfram, Walt and Marcia Whiteman. "The Role of Dialect Interference in Composition." ERIC Document ED 045971, 1971.

Wolfram, Walt and Ralph Fasold. "Social Dialects and Education." *Sociolinguistic Aspects of Language Learning and Teaching*. Ed. J.B. Pride. London: Oxford University Press, 1979.

Part II
CLINICAL AND PROFESSIONAL IMPLICATIONS

Chapter IV

SOCIAL DIALECTS AND THE SPEECH-LANGUAGE CLINICIAN:

An Overview of Clinical and Professional Issues

NICHOLAS G. BOUNTRESS

MANY critical and sensitive issues have perplexed the educational establishment of the United States throughout its history, but few have created more controversy, rancor and debate than those related to the education of culturally and ethnically diverse populations, in particular black children from the lower socioeconomic level. The most common areas of concern have been related to black children's demonstrated inability to perform at levels equivalent to caucasian children in academic settings and on formal tests of intellectual and scholastic abilities. Historically, the response of educators has been to engage in racially-based tracking, the procedure by which "educationally disadvantaged" children are placed in academic groupings with similar children who are assumed to have a lowered capacity for learning. Such grouping has frequently stimulated the attitude on the part of teachers that lower academic track children are non-achievers from whom little can be expected academically, an attitude which leads to further academic failure and increased drop-out rates from the nation's schools by many minority children. Educational researchers have suggested that such children fail because of genetic and environmental factors which supposedly operate within "disadvantaged" populations. In short, when black children failed in the public schools, it was because of genetic inferiority or the lack of environmental stimulation, factors with which the schools felt they were powerless to contend. Much of the support for these conclusions and attitudes was found in studies which investigated the linguistic abilities of lower socioeconomic level, and frequently black, children as compared with the linguistic abilities of middle- and upper-class, and frequently, white children. Because linguistic abilities were equated with intellectual capacity and because lower socieconomic-level children typically fared worse than their middle- and upper-class counterparts on linguistic tasks, lower socioeconomic-level children were often regarded as being intellectually inferior.

The above-mentioned studies, which formed the basis for what is regarded as the "language deficit" position, focused upon four major linguistic parameters: vocabulary, speech-sound development, mean length of response, and speech-sound discrimination. Illustrative of the vocabulary studies are those of Carson and Rabin (1960), John (1963) and M. Deutsch (1965), the former utilizing the Ammons and Ammons Full-Range Picture Vocabulary Test (1958) and the latter two using the Peabody Picture Vocabulary Test (Dunn and Dunn, 1965). In all three cases, lower socioeconomic-level and/or black subjects performed poorly when compared to middle-class and/or white subjects. Examples of studies of speech-sound development are those of Irwin (1948), Templin (1957), Raph (1967) and Andersland (1961). Irwin's research indicated that infants from laboring class backgrounds developed speech sounds at a slower rate than did middle-class children, while Templin found a similar tendency among children aged three to eight years. Raph found that children enrolled in a Head Start program made numerous articulation errors, while Andersland found the same tendency among lower class kindergarten children. Studies of mean length of response by Templin (1957), Lawton (1964), and Hess and Shipman (1965) typify the "language deficit" research that indicated a marked tendency for black and lower-class children to use more abbreviated and monosyllabic responses than middle-class children. Hess and Shipman, in particular, noted that mothers of black children engaged in fewer lengthy conversations and stimulated shorter responses from their children than did the mothers of white children. Two studies which are frequently cited regarding the speech-sound discrimination deficits of economically-disadvantaged children are those of C. Deutsch (1964) and Clark and Richards (1966), both of which utilized the Wepman Test of Auditory Discrimination (1958). Deutsch suggested that such deficits were a result of the selective "tuning-out" process of the reticular formation of inner city children, while Clark and Richards believed that the parents of these children were less likely to stress attentiveness to verbal cues than were the parents of middle-class children.

Studies of this nature which buttressed the "language deficit" position held by many educators and researchers persisted into the 1960's. However, soon after the publication of Chomsky's (1964) perspectives regarding linguistic theory, research of a significantly different design and intent was initiated by linguists in the major urban areas of the United States. Eschewing the tendency of the "language deficit" researchers to engage in comparative studies of black and white and middle- and lower-class children using white, middle class-normed tests, these researchers analyzed the phonological and syntactic variations produced by black children and described those variations in terms of linguistic rules. In so doing, Labov (1975), Wolfram (1969), McDavid (1970), Fasold and Wolfram (1972), Stewart (1964), and others, often described as dialectal variations those characteristics which earlier "language deficit" researchers had described as aberrant. Of particular consequence was that a corpus of rule-governed linguistic characteristics was identified which was common to "black English" speakers regardless of geographical area. While this research indicated that dialect speakers in a specific locale did not use these characteristics exclusively, and, in fact, often used regional variations which were observed in other American dialects, the features described were found to be used in varying degrees by most blacks from the lower socioeconomic level. The most important implication of this research was that it provided evidence which indicated that black English is a complex, consistent, and rule-governed system, and not deficient and haphazard as "language deficit" researchers had noted. It was this body of information and this perspective which formed the basis for the "language different" hypothesis.

While the urban language studies were of significant importance for the profession of speech-language pathology, it is difficult to ascertain whether that research has had a major impact on the manner in which clinicians structure intervention programs for black children from the lower socioeconomic level. It is likely that the impact was, at least, theoretical in that most clinicians are conversant with the "language difference — language deficit" argument and can identify certain commonly-occurring dialectal characteristics. However, as Taylor (1979) has indicated, the appropriate diagnosis of and speech-language intervention with black populations is compounded by the persistent use of linguistically-biased standardized tests and therapeutic methodologies which are not culturally sensitive. In short, Taylor's conclusions suggest that not even the most basic questions have been answered regarding clinical management of communication disorders in blacks. Wolfram (1979) indicated that basic issues regarding evaluation and treatment of dialect speakers are of constant and recurring concern among clinicians. Bountress (1980), in a study regarding the attitudes and professional training of clinicians providing services to black populations, found that speech-language clinicians felt ill-equipped to differentially diagnose dialectal variations from pathological variations. While the clinicians in the study were aware of the importance of the pertinent theoretical issues, they felt that their academic training was insufficient to aid them in the practical matters of differential diagnosis and the prescribing and developing of intervention programs.

In 1969, Baratz published an article in which she examined a number of critical questions concerned with professional service delivery by educators to dialect speakers. Specifically, Baratz inquired as to who should provide what services as well as when and why (Baratz, 1969). It would appear that, given some of the concerns of Taylor, Wolfram, Bountress and others and the fact that such concerns have persisted for more than a decade after the major urban language studies, an examination of Baratz' questions still has relevance, if not urgency, for the speech-language clinician. It will be the purpose of the following discussion to examine these concerns, specifically with regard to the roles and responsibilities of the clinician and in light of some of the more recent research by professionals in both the fields of sociolinguistics and speech-language pathology.

WHY IS INTERVENTION NECESSARY
WITH DIALECT SPEAKERS?

Education in the United States has been described as having numerous and varied goals, but among the most traditionally-espoused and respected have been that schools should maximize the potential of and intellectually stimulate and guide students from all cultural and economic backgrounds. The ultimate purposes of such goals are to prepare students to take their places as productive members of society and to have all citizens participate in the economic mainstream of that society. If education is to fulfill its promise, any barriers to those goals must be identified and eliminated. An important issue which must be examined with regard to dialect speakers is whether there are barriers which interfere with the educational process and the attainment of the above goals for persons who do not use the standard dialect of the school, and, if so, what the barriers are that presently exist. As was noted previously, the high frequency of academic failure and disproportionate drop-out rate of lower socioeconomic-level black children, many of whom are speakers of non-standard English, indicates that there are significant problems which have never been resolved. The nature of those problems, however, has been the source of much conflictory debate and conjecture. A review of the research of Blank and Solomon (1969), Caplan and Ruble (1964), Cohn (1959) and numerous others suggests that the initial barrier which minority, particularly black, children must face in the schools is having to adjust to the fact that classroom activities are transacted in standard English. The principal problem which was generally presumed to be operational was that the linguistic interference created by the differences between native and school dialects results in comprehension difficulty for the child, causing him to miss or misinterpret portions of the information transmitted by the classroom teacher. However, the later research of Frentz (1971), Ramsey (1972) and others, which examined black children's comprehension of both Black English and standard English stimuli, indicates otherwise. The results of these studies indicated that dialect speakers have no significant difficulty in the comprehension of standard English. It was also a widely-held belief that, as suggested in the "language-deficit" studies, the restricted and flawed oral language expression of black children was reflective of inferior intellectual capacity, a factor which predestined these children to academic failure. However, given the results and conclusions of the major urban language studies, it is apparent that no such widespread deficiencies of language occur within black populations. Furthermore, it is the concensus of modern linguists, as expressed by the Linguistic Society of America (1972), that the minimal ability needed to learn and to speak a human language or dialect requires a high order of native intelligence. The very fact that the measurement of human intelligence is so inexact makes the conclusions concerning intelligence reached by deficit theorists particularly ill-conceived. If, then, it is not subnormal intelligence and linguistic abilities which predispose dialect speakers as a group to academic failure, what factors do play a more central role in this dilemma? There is sufficient reason to believe that these factors are related to the socio-cultural confrontation which occurs when the child's culture meets and clashes with the school culture. As Loban (1968) has stated, language and social caste are inextricably interwoven, and the language of the black child from the lower socioeconomic level reflects that lower status. The child whose awareness of his inferior class status is accentuated by his awareness of his language difference may demonstrate a reticence to participate, even if he is relatively apt at decoding and encoding the classroom dialect. Furthermore, the child is faced with the serious practical dilemma of how to orally respond in class. Does he use "home language" and risk possible disparagement by the teacher, attempt "school language" and risk the likely ridicule of his cultural peers, or avoid either punishment by remaining mute, or, at most, monosyllabic? Given the massive number of studies which describe the lack of verbosity of such children, it is likely that the latter option is a common choice. However, the child who is able to overcome his reticence to speak in class must also overcome the barriers posed by teacher attitudes. Cohn (1959) stated that class-antagonism on the part of the middleclass teacher is one of the most important contributing factors in the alienation of lower-class children from our schools. That antagonism can be most effectively transmitted through the teacher's verbal and non-verbal responses to the black child's language. If the unwary or insensitive teacher criticizes, ridicules or harshly corrects the child's language, it may discourage attempts at further communication and severely damage the child's self-concept. Furthermore, if the teacher perceives nonstandard dialects as being deficient and, therefore, indicative of lowered intelligence, that fact may be communicated to the dialect speaker who fulfills his teacher's expectations of failure.

Early intervention is necessary to reduce the chance, or at least the frequency, of such negative interactions, and to prepare the child for survival, adjustment, and success in the middle-class school environment. All too often, negative teacher attitudes and expectations and the child's reticence to respond and his discomfort in what may be perceived as an alien atmosphere may cause him to perform below the level of his middle-class peers. Constant failure and frustration create conditions to which very few children can adjust, with the result being a marked tendency for lower socioeconomic-level blacks to drop out of school altogether. Such an occurrence is a critical link in what Williams (1970) refers to as the "poverty cycle" in which economic disadvantage begets educational advantage which begets employment disadvantage which maintains economic disadvantage. The school's purpose should be to arrest the cycle within its own domain and, ideally, increase the potential employability of the child from the lower socioeconomic level thereby increasing the probability of economic success. This purpose can only be accomplished if the school ensures the fact that the child will not drop out before graduation, and this can only occur if classroom teachers, administrators, and all other educational personnel are sensitive to the cultural and linguistic backgrounds of each child. Most critically, educators must create an atmosphere in which the child feels free to express himself without overt or covert penalty. This can be greatly facilitated if educators understand that nonstandard dialects, including Black English, are as complex and as reflective of intellectual capability as standard dialects. To not appreciate these fundamental concerns and act accordingly will prolong the poverty cycle by assuring the failure of high school dropouts who have little chance of competing for jobs in a high technology era with less-than-basic skills.

While decreasing the number of lower socioeconomic-level black children who drop out of school is a formidable task, it is only a beginning. It is also imperative that the child learn those basic skills which will allow for greater marketability after graduation, in particular reading and oral communication skills. Wolfram (1979), Labov

(1975) and others have indicated that reading problems encountered by dialect speakers are less likely to be caused by dialectal interference than by the cultural conflict of the school and home cultures. Therefore, it is likely that progress in reading will be best facilitated by teacher sensitivity to the child's culture as well as by an understanding by the teacher and child of interdialectal variations. While the preceding can also serve as valuable aids in the teaching of oral communication skills, there has been frequent debate over which pedagogy to employ. Some educators have suggested that the child be allowed to continue to use his native dialect, because it allows for the maintenance of cultural integrity and self-concept. However, others suggest that standard English should be taught because, as has been noted earlier in this discussion, it affords the opportunity for greater success, or at least results in less penalty, in the school. It has also been suggested that, just as the use of standard English allows for easier passage through the schools, it may allow for greater accessibility to desirable employment opportunities. One of the few studies to examine this hypothesis was conducted by Terrell and Terrell (1983). The authors selected six black female university students who posed as applicants for secretarial positions. Three students were Black English speakers and three were standard English speakers. One hundred job interview situations were eventually selected for the purposes of gathering data, with none including black or female interviewers. Each student went to a job interview with bogus credentials, a tape recorder, and a stop-watch to record the length of the session. The results of the Terrells' study indicated that interviewers spent a significantly greater amount of time with the standard English speakers, which was assumed to be a measure of the interviewers' interest in the applicant, and offered the standard English speakers a significantly greater number of jobs. It was also observed that the Black English speakers were more frequently offered jobs at lower wage levels. While this study requires duplication and validation, it offers interesting insights into a matter about which there has, heretofore, been only speculation. If its underlying hypothesis is valid, it will provide further verification of the need for early intervention with dialect speakers to prevent the maintenance of employment and economic disadvantages which are part of the poverty cycle.

As important as the arguments and concerns have been with re-

gard to the need for intervention with dialect speakers before the deleterious effects of educational failure and employment disadvantage
occur, there is a need for more forceful advocacy. Specifically, there
has been a need for well-considered legislation which can focus upon
the issues of bidialectal education, prescribe changes in the educational system, and generate sufficient national interest so that the results will be disseminated by the media. One of the few acts of
legislation to have such an impact was a federal suit filed in Michigan's Eastern District Court during the summer of 1979. The final
disposition of "Martin Luther King Elementary School Children et
al, Plaintiffs, v. Ann Arbor School District, Defendant" has come to
be regarded as the "Ann Arbor decision" and has provided a
precedent-establishing rationale for the recognition of the validity of
non-standard English as well as for stipulating some of the responsibilities of school systems. The suit was initiated by black parents and
their attorneys who claimed that the children's use of dialect inter-
fered with their equal participation in academic programs. In particular, the plaintiffs claimed that the school had failed to recognize the
pervasive use of dialect and failed to understand its influence upon
the teaching of reading and standard English. Furthermore, it was
the plaintiff's contention that the school's failure to respond appropriately resulted in students' lack of normal progress in academic
subjects and often led to inappropriate grade placement. The basis
for much of the parents' argument was provided by a team of experts
comprised of linguists and educators who discussed the current state
of knowledge regarding Black English. Apart from providing examples of the characteristic features of the dialect, the experts discussed
the embarassment and shame which dialect speakers feel regarding
their language when confronted by a critical teacher. While such
negative reactions were described as impeding the learning process
in general, they were described as exerting a particularly profound
influence upon the process of learning to read standard English.
Specifically, it was noted that children, when confronted with negative teacher attitudes and the task of reading in a different dialect,
may reject efforts to teach them to read. It was observed that the resultant inability to read can affect children's success in other academic areas as well.

On the basis of the information provided him, Judge Charles
Joiner concluded that, while the teachers at King School had not

treated the children's dialect as inferior, they did not take it into account when teaching the children to read standard English. In the opinion of Judge Joiner, failing to consider the influence of the home language creates a language barrier to the learning of standard English which may ultimately be the source of reading problems. In his judicial response, he directed the defendant to submit a plan which would help the King School teachers identify Black English and to use that information to develop a program for teaching students to read standard English. The plan which the Ann Arbor Board of Education submitted to the court included a Formal Instructional Component, and a Classroom Application Component, as well as a new reading program component utilizing the Houghton-Mifflin basal reading series. The Formal Instructional Component included twenty hours of formal instruction for the teachers by a team of language arts consultants, while the Classroom Application Component incorporated the use of the instructional content in classroom settings. The objectives of the instructional component were as follows:

a. recognize generally the basic features of a language system as they apply to dialect differences.

b. be able to describe in general the concept of a dialect and dialect differences within the English language.

c. be sensitive to the value judgments about dialect differences which people often make and communicate to others.

d. be able to describe the basic linguistic features of Black English as it contrasts with standard English.

e. show appreciation for the history and background of Black English.

f. recognize readily children and adults speaking the Black English dialect.

g. be able to identify without prompting the specific linguistic features by which they recognized a speaker of Black English dialect.

h. be able to discuss knowledgeably the important linguistic issues in code-switching between Black English and standard written English.

i. be able to identify possible instructional strategies that can be used to aid children in code-switching between Black English and standard English.

j. use miscue analysis strategies to distinguish between a dialect shift and a decoding mistake when analyzing an oral reading sample.

k. be able to describe a variety of language experience activities that can be used to complement the linguistic basal reader program.

Labov (1981) has indicated that the Ann Arbor decision was of extraordinary importance because it represented the initiatives of black scholars and black linguists and because it represented the climax of a fifteen-year struggle to legitimize the notion of Black English. Perhaps of ultimate practical importance is that, as Labov notes, it has provided an impressive rationale for intervention with non-standard English speakers. Specifically, it has alerted educators to the fact that the courts will intervene in cases where the schools are not sensitive to the barriers to learning standard English faced by minority groups. Indicative of this latter point is a related class action suit reported by Hechinger (1979) in which parents of black and Hispanic children enrolled in New York schools complained that their children had been incorrectly diagnosed and placed in special classes. A federal judge found for the plaintiffs and ordered the school system to re-evaluate all children in the special schools as well as to develop a training program to improve procedures by which children were to be identified and placed.

The Ann Arbor decision and cases similar to that described above by Hechinger have significant implications for the speech-language clinician, as well as for the special educator. Paramount among these is that accurate intervention is necessary with dialect speakers so that misdiagnosis and inappropriate placement can be avoided. Specifically, speech-language clinicians and special educators must be able to differentiate between language differences, as exemplified by nonstandard dialects, and actual pathological linguistic variations. The critical purpose of such differentiation is to ensure that a dialect speaker who is speech-language disordered, learning disabled, or mildly retarded will be enrolled in a remedial program which is appropriate and beneficial for his needs. Conversely, for legal, ethical, and humanitarian reasons, it is vital that the dialect speaker who does not demonstrate these problems not be enrolled in such program. While these points appear to be highly obvious in theory, they are considerably less so when theory is linked with practice. For example, as Taylor (1980) has observed, while some studies indicate that the incidence of speech-language disorders among blacks may be as much as two to three times as high as that for whites, other studies that use procedures which are reflective of cultural and linguistic norms indicate considerably lower incidence figures. The critical variable in such matters is the sensitivity of the diagnostic instrument, as well as the examiner, in recognizing the difference between those items and tasks which are linguistically and culturally biased and those which are not. It is obvious that many instruments and procedures are not culturally sensitive in this manner, and that the reason for the failure of large numbers of black children on tests of reading, writing, vocabulary, academic achievement, intelligence, and speech and language owes to this fact. Such diagnostic methodology reflects the common proclivity to adhere to standards of correctness which are blind to the linguistic variations, attitudes, values, perceptions, and environment of non-white, non-middle-class populations. The ultimate tragedy of these erroneous procedures is that children are misdiagnosed and placed in educational and remedial settings which are inappropriate for their specific learning needs. While no actual figures are available on the extent of erroneous placement, Dunn (1968), a past president of the Council for Exceptional Children, has inferred that those figures may be extremely high. Dunn indicated that over one-third of all special educators in the United States are teachers of the mentally retarded, and that sixty to eighty percent of their pupils are from low socioeconomic backgrounds. Dunn and Mercer (1973) agree that this population, the majority of which is labeled as being educable mentally retarded, is frequently placed on the basis of low scores on standardized tests without reference to the sociolinguistic or cultural reasons for such depressed performance. Obviously, such problems are not found solely in the domain of the special educator. In a recent study by Bountress and Hayes (1982) of ninety-three black children who had been referred for further testing on the basis of failure on the Fluharty Preschool Speech and Language Screening Test (1974), at least eight percent would not have been referred had regional dialectal variations not been scored as errors. As a result, valuable diagnostic time was wasted on follow-up testing and, more critically, erroneous educational placement occurred.

While the humanitarian issues related to the incorrect assessment and placement of children who are dialect speakers should obviously be foremost in the minds of speech-language clinicians and other professionals who work with handicapped populations, there are also legal issues which cannot be overlooked. In particular, Public Law 94-142 provides a significant rationale for attending closely to matters of intervention with speakers of nonstandard English. For the purpose of protecting the child against inappropriate evaluation procedures, P.L. 94-142 mandates that "testing and evaluation materials and procedures used for the purposes of evaluation and placement of handicapped children must be selected so as not to be racially or culturally discriminatory." Furthermore, with regard to placement procedures, P.L. 94-142 mandates that each public agency must draw upon information from a variety of sources, including the child's social or cultural background. Given the likelihood that many of the testing and evaluation procedures of speech-language clinicians and special educators are both racially and culturally discriminatory and that resultant placement is likely to be in non-compliance with P.L. 94-142's directive that such placements be in the least restrictive and most appropriate environment, it is truly surprising that lawsuits have not been more commonplace.

The issue of why intervention is necessary with dialect speakers is, therefore, complex and multi-faceted. Intervention programs are essential to stem the academic failure of minority groups in educational settings and reduce the frequency of high school drop-outs, to increase the potential for improved educational, employment, and economic opportunity, and to assure compliance with legal mandates. Speech-language clinicians should become particularly aware of their role in the intervention process and the necessity for developing and using culture-fair diagnostic procedures as well as for structuring programs which reflect a sensitivity to cultural diversity.

WHO SHOULD STRUCTURE INTERVENTION
PROGRAMS FOR DIALECT SPEAKERS?

Among the many researchers who work provided data-based and philosophical support for the language-deficit hypothesis, few have been more influential than Basil Bernstein and Arthur Jensen.

While their arguments were at opposite sides of the continuum on the subject, with Bernstein advocating the critical role of environment and social codes in the language of lower socioeconomic-level children and Jensen the role of genetic factors in the intellectual characteristics of blacks, both presented forceful contemporary arguments which were popular for significant periods of time. In fact, residual influence of these arguments still persists through the present day. Bernstein (1965) described the working class child's family environment and peer relationships as factors which led to reduced verbal exploration and elaboration and which ultimately led to the child's use of a "restricted" language code. This code was said to be characterized by fewer syntactic and lexical alternatives than standard English and created an inability to facilitate the "verbal expansion of the speaker's intent." In later writings, Bernstein (1970) indicated that the child's use of a restricted code does not mean that he is linguistically deprived, but that it does limit the child's orientation to "universalistic orders of meaning." In any event, it was Bernstein's description of restricted codes and its association with working class children which was frequently cited in the literature that promoted the language-deficit hypothesis. Jensen (1969), on the other hand, argued that genetic factors are more important than environmental factors with regard to intelligence and scholastic achievement, and that real average differences in intellectual ability exist between groups. Jensen also noted that, because intelligence tests measure higher mental processes and a review of results from such tests indicates that blacks score approximately one standard deviation below whites, significant differences exist between blacks and whites with regard to mental abilities. As a result of such differences, compensatory education programs fail because they cannot narrow the genetically-based gap between black and white children. These arguments gave particular credence to the arguments of many language-deficit proponents that the disordered language of black children was a reflection of reduced intellectual abilities.

In retrospect, the most glaring problem with the arguments of Bernstein and Jensen was that they were made in a vacuum. Information of a most sensitive and potentially damaging nature that affected the education and well-being of large numbers of persons was disseminated without the consideration of and consultation with professionals from other disciplines who could have provided additional valuable insights. This is not to demean the role which sociologists and educational psychologists can play in the educational adjustment of minority children, but to suggest that there are other professionals who, by their training and experience, have a better technical understanding of the nature of language and its relationship to intelligence. For example, in contrast to the statements of Bernstein are the linguistic arguments and evidence supplied by Labov (1970), among others, which indicate that an examination of the language of working-class children reveals rule-governed grammatical structure as well as logic and verbosity which are the equal of middle-class speakers. In contrast to the statements of both Bernstein and Jensen are the conclusions of the Linguistic Society of America (1972) that non-standard dialects of English are neither conceptually nor logically inadequate, and that they contain all the grammatical structure necessary for logical thought. Furthermore, it has been through the efforts of linguists, speech-language pathologists and other professionals that the validity of standardized tests as acceptable and culturally-fair measures of speech, language, and intelligence has been called into serious question.

The limitations of the research of Bernstein and Jensen serve to underscore the fact that no single discipline should consider itself to be the sole repository of knowledge that is pertinent to educational intervention with dialect-speaking minority children. As has been discussed, there are not only linguistic and educational factors which must be considered, but also sociological, psychological, anthropological, and psychometric considerations as well. As Bronstein (1973) has discussed, sociolinguists have professional origins which can be traced to disciplines concerned with these areas as well as English and foreign languages and have a crucial role in the intervention process. While anthropologists may have been among the earliest professionals to investigate the linguistic systems of social groups, it has been sociolinguists who have engaged in the most intensive research in that field during the past two decades. Of critical importance has been the sociolinguist's study of linguistic structure as a function of social strata and cultural and ethnic background. More than any other specialist, the sociolinguist has studied the interaction of social setting and social identity of the speaker and of the receiver, phenomena which are fundamental to an understanding of linguistic diversity. However, it should not be overlooked that numerous other professionals have critical roles to play in the process of educational intervention with dialect speakers. Such professionals are not only of critical importance for the manner in which they interpret and apply sociolinguistic research, but also for those unique contributions which are reflective of their disciplines' particular areas of expertise. Taylor (1980), for example, cites the role of professionals in the fields of intercultural and interpersonal communication who can facilitate interaction between persons of diverse backgrounds. Shuy (1971) has long stressed the role of university teacher-training programs in preparing future professionals through the inclusion of classes in the nature of language, language variations, and the teaching of standard English. The role of the classroom teacher is obviously of critical importance, not only in didactic activities, but also in facilitating the child's adjustment to the school environment. As illustrated by the Ann Arbor decision, this role becomes all the more important when the teacher has an understanding of non-standard English as well as the potential for interference of the native dialect in reading, speaking, and writing the standard dialect in the school. The roles played by sociologists, anthropologists and psychologists are relevant because it is through these disciplines which other professionals can gain insight into social and cultural influences, the nature of community and familial organization, the effects of poverty upon children's aspirations and academic performance, and related issues of importance.

The role of the speech-language clinician in intervention with dialect speakers has been gradually evolving during the past two decades, with the greatest changes in the description of the breadth of that role occurring since the early 1970's. Prior to that time, speech-language clinicians tended to approach dialectal variations as deficiencies and enrolled dialect speakers in therapy for correction of what were perceived to be phonological and syntactic errors. With the revolutionary urban language studies in the late 1960's and early 1970's came the realization that clinicians needed to become cognizant of the linguistic and cultural biases of their diagnostic instruments and wary of which children they were diagnosing as speech-language disordered. A message which was inferred from the sociolinguistic studies was that matters of language differences were better left to remedial English teachers and linguists. However, it became readily apparent that professional collaboration in educational intervention with dialect speakers was not only warranted but vital. As McDavid (1970) emphasized, no single talent is all-sufficient and the clinician and remedial English teacher need to cooperate with linguists, neurologists, psychologists, and others. McDavid noted that information from these specialists should be in the hands of clinicians and that the clinician should be an important educational resource, particularly in cases of stuttering, cleft palate, and neurological language disorder where the expertise of the linguist may only be of peripheral importance. However, a movement for the expanded role of the clinician in cases of social dialects also began to emanate from within the professional ranks of speech-language pathologists during the 1970's, and continued into the 1980's. While the clinician's primary role with minority populations was initially envisaged as including the differential diagnosis of pathological from different language variations, and the subsequent structuring of culturally-sensitive therapy approaches for those diagnosed as being language delayed or disordered, speech-language pathologists such as Adler (1971), Williams (1972), Baskervill (1977), Bountress (1980b), Eisenson & Ogilvie (1983) and others have suggested that the clinician has other roles to play as well. Baskervill, and Eisenson & Ogilvie, for example, advocate the function of the clinician as a resource consultant to the classroom teacher. Principal responsibilities of this role would include helping the teacher to identify regional differences in pronunciation and grammar, to identify the linguistic and cultural biases of achievement and intelligence tests, and to structure programs to promote increased motivation to verbalize as well as to learn the standard dialect of the school. Given the mandates of Public Law 94-142 that define the role of the clinician in terms of speech-language impairment, the preceding description as resource consultant and advocate for the culturally different child would appear to be both appropriate and reasonable.

Some speech-language pathologists, however, have advocated a role which goes beyond the traditionally-defined responsibilities of the clinician. Adler (1971), Williams (1972), and Bountress (1980b) have noted that the principal barrier to providing services to dialect speakers may have less to do with professional competency than with professional perspective. The conceptual model which clinincians have used has been defined too narrowly by professionals themselves as well as by the American Speech-Language-Hearing Association.

There is a need for clinicians to change this model so that they can not only correct the truly pathological linguistic variations of dialect-speakers but also teach standard English to persons with different linguistic patterns. Williams has maintained that the speech-language pathologist is the professional who is best-suited for such a role because of a traditional clinical aptitude for applying knowledge to practical questions. Furthermore, the days when university training programs in speech-language pathology gave only a casual consideration to linguistic theory are long since over. Clinicians who have been trained during the past decade are not only familiar with psycholinguistic and sociolinguistic research but other behavioral sciences research related to the structuring of intervention programs for persons from a variety of socioeconomic backgrounds.

Despite the logic and eloquence of the arguments posed by Adler, Williams and others, as well as the progress made by university training programs in focusing upon the practical as well as theoretical issues related to non-standard dialects, there has been a reluctance on the part of speech-language clinicians to serve as resource consultants in the schools as well as to teach standard English to dialect speakers outside of the school setting. While this reluctance may be due to the time restrictions imposed by traditional responsibilities, it may be that a great deal of the profession's reticence is due to the fact that the American Speech-Language-Hearing Association (ASHA) has not, until recently, delineated the role of the clinician with regard to social dialects. However, in an acknowledgement of the issues raised by the above researchers, ASHA published a position paper on social dialects in 1983 which represents an important step in the profession's delivery of services to non-standard English speakers. While noting that the professional priority of clinicians is to serve the "truly communicatively handicapped," the position paper stated that the speech-language pathologist may also provide elective clinical services to non-standard English speakers who do not present a disorder. In these cases, the clinician's goal should be to teach standard English while respecting the native dialect. The clinical requisites cited are knowledge of dialectal features, contrastive analysis procedures, and the effects of attitudes toward dialects. The professional implications and practical effect of this statement remain to be seen, but it can be hoped that ASHA's sanctioning of the above activities will motivate clinicians to play a more active consultative role in assisting teachers who teach dialect speakers and stimulate the development of quality intervention programs for minority populations.

A final issue regarding who should provide services to dialect speakers is that of race. Specifically, is it more beneficial for the purposes and results of intervention that the Black English speaker be placed with a black professional, or, in the case of speech-language intervention, a black clinician? The largest body of literature on the topic is found in the fields of sociology and psychology and examines the influence of racial experimenter effects upon children's performance on a variety of tasks. Much of this research has suggested that black children perform poorly for white examiners because they consciously inhibit hostile feelings, thereby interfering with spontaneous cognitive functioning. It is also suggested that the presence of a white examiner who will pass judgment on their adequacy strengthens black children's self-derogatory attitude and expectations of failure. While much of the research takes this type of negative interaction for granted, it also suggests that the issue may be more complex than black-white interaction only. Such variables as task content, instructional set, geographical location, and attitudes, age, sex, and socioeconomic status of the examiner may play crucial roles. It should also be observed that many of the studies of racial experimenter effects are marred by methodological inadequacies and inconsistent findings, particularly with regard to intelligence and personality testing and psychotherapeutic interaction. One of the few studies in the field of speech-language pathology which has dealt with this topic was conducted by Bountress and Bountress (1982) who investigated the role of experimenter effects on the measurement of mean length of utterance (MLU). Utilizing a test-retest, black-white alternating examiner design, twenty-one black and twenty-one white children were tested by a team of black and white undergraduate university students. Each child was engaged in conversation twice, once by a black clinician and once by a white clinician. MLU's were computed and compared with reference to the race of the examiner and the child who was tested. The results indicated no significant differences in MLU as a function of race. While studies of this nature are in need of replication and extension to a wider range of speech-language activities, the implication is that race may not be as critical a variable in clinical activity as the early research in sociology and psychology has suggested. It may be that such fundamental factors as the clinician's cultural sensitivity, personal and social attributes and professional expertise are of more profound significance than the race of either the child or the clinician. In fact, as Baratz (1969) has observed in the teaching of standard English to Black English speakers, there is no assurance that black teachers will be any more sensitive to ghetto speech and ghetto speakers than will white teachers. Perhaps the wisest statement regarding this issue is that by the National Urban League's Whitney Young, as cited by Adler (1971), who concluded that the black population is more concerned with the quality of service than the race of the helping person.

WHAT INTERVENTION PROCEDURES ARE APPROPRIATE FOR DIALECT SPEAKERS?

As evidenced by the American Speech-Language — Hearing Association's position statement on social dialects, there has been a feeling among many speech-language pathologists that their role with dialect-speaking minority populations has needed clearer definition. Specifically, there has been a need to decide whether or not it is within the purview of the clinician to teach standard English to persons who present language differences. The ASHA position reflects the attitude of a number of professionals in the field who believe that the clinician has a critical function which, while focused upon the facilitation of linguistic change, has as its ultimate purposes the successful adjustment to the school environment and the providing of access to greater economic opportunity by minority individuals. The decision to develop intervention procedures for dialect speakers entails, as has been noted by numerous writers, more than the obligation to provide additional services, but requires the cultivation of a non-traditional clinical perspective. Such a perspective requires a new theoretical framework for decisions concerning intervention and resultant changes in the procedures used in the intervention process. Regarding this theoretical framework for decision-making, the clinician must first examine the variety of options available in teaching spoken English and then select that option which is most appropriate for the needs of the child. Wolfram and

Fasold (1974) have suggested that there are four such conceivable options. One option is to teach standard English but eradicate all vestiges of the native dialect; a second option is to eradicate the native dialect, but not explicitly teach standard English; a third option is to teach standard English while allowing retention of the native dialect; a fourth option is allowing retention of the native dialect without teaching standard English. As Wolfram and Fasold indicate, the second goal may be considered to be nonsense because it infers that the child is left with neither his own dialect or the standard dialect. The fourth option is highly controversial in that it advocates the retention of the native dialect while attacking the negative language attitudes of persons who are in positions of power. At the core of this argument is the valid contention that non-standard dialects are legitimate, rule-governed systems. Therefore, it is the role of institutions to alter their prejudicial attitudes and not the responsibility of minority populations to change their different but not deficient language patterns. Despite the validity of this argument's underlying assumption, it is unfortunate but true that it has proven to be easier to alter a child's language than it has been to make changes in negative institutional attitudes. With the stakes being the educational adjustment of the child, with its consequences of later economic survival, it would seem that this argument may be more appropriate in a future less-imperfect society.

The first and third options discussed by Wolfram and Fasold represent the teaching goals which have been hotly debated by the language-deficit and language-different advocates. The first option is underscored by a belief in the deficiency of non-standard dialects, with its translation into educational practice exemplified by programs which eradicate the native dialect and supplant it with standard English. Until relatively recently, this was the option exercised by many speech-language clinicians. The third option, which is advocated by most contemporary linguists, is supportive of the position of bidialectalism, or, teaching the student to use standard English but not eradicating the native dialect. This option is based upon belief in the legitimacy of the native dialect as well as an acceptance of its use. The educational objective of bidialectal programs is to have the child use either the standard or nonstandard dialect as the situation demands.

Given the position of the American Speech-Language-Hearing

Association with regard to social dialects, as well as the research of sociolinguists during the past two decades, it is obvious that the non-traditional clinical perspective which speech-language pathologists need to develop in working with dialect speakers must embrace bi-dialectalism. As the preceding discussion implied, such an approach to the delivery of services is a radical departure from the traditional role of the clinician. Rather than correcting pathological syntactic and phonological variations, the clinician must accept the non-standard productions while facilitating the learning of standard English by comparing and contrasting the rules of the one dialect with the other. However, the learning of the methodology is only one of several changes which the clinician must make when redirecting his efforts from correcting communication disorders to facilitating bi-dialectal proficiency. In particular, the clinician must be prepared to aid classroom teachers and other professionals in relating to and teaching dialect speakers, as well as in describing dialectal variations and their role in standardized test biases. There is also a great necessity for becoming highly attuned to the sensitivity of parents whose children are enrolled in bidialectal instructional programs, and in gauging and acting upon these parents' attitudes regarding the relevancy of such programs. There is an urgent need for ongoing examination of diagnostic tools and assessment procedures so that accurate differential diagnosis of deficiencies from differences can occur and appropriate and culture-sensitive programs can be constructed. The following discussion provides an overview of these issues in the context of the role of the speech-language clinician.

Diagnosis

The basis of appropriate and effective educational intervention with dialect speakers, as with any population, lies with appropriate and effective diagnosis. For the speech-language clinician, diagnosis should clearly differentiate between the dialect speaker who has pathological linguistic variations and the dialect speaker who does not. Such a differentiation allows the clinician to develop a plan of therapy, or correction, for the speaker using pathological variations or a program to promote the learning of standard English for the dialect speaker whose language is consistent with and reflective of his native linguistic community. Unfortunately, the traditional tools used by speech-language clinicians have not allowed for this clear differentiation, a fact underscored by Adler (1979), Taylor (1980), Bountress and Hayes (1982), and numerous others. All too frequently, the inherent linguistic and cultural biases of these tools have led to the misdiagnosis of language differences as deficits, with the biases for the most part being attributable to the use of middle-class normative standards. The problems posed for non-middle-class populations who are administered these tests are many and, as reviewed by Adler (1979), may be nonlinguistic as well as linguistic. For example, the stimuli presented, the strategies needed, and the responses expected may be outside the experience of the minority child. The verbal styles required by the test are likely to be considered correct only if they are the styles typically used by middle-class children. Differing semantic, syntactic, and phonological stimuli may create confusion and reticence in dialect-speaking children, and the use of standard English responses as criteria for correctness will typically cause these children's verbal responses to be judged as inadequate. Finally, a factor which requires more careful scrutiny is the test situation itself. The atmosphere and structure of the testing experience have been conjectured to be less familiar to and comfortable for the lower-class child. While the validity of this latter concern is open to some debate, one is reminded of the interviews conducted by Labov (1970) with black youths from New York City. While the subjects responded with unelaborated, perfunctory, and monosyllabic utterances to both black and white interviewers in formal settings, their responses were extended, detailed and spontaneous when they were interviewed under less formal and antiseptic circumstances.

While the results of surprisingly few studies have been published or disseminated to clinicians regarding the linguistic and cultural biases of speech and language tests which are used, those which have been presented indicate that the biases are pervasive. Among the earliest examinations of this subject was that by Wolfram, Williams, and Taylor (1972) which focused upon the Northwestern Syntax Screening Test (NSST) (Lee, 1971), the Wepman Auditory Discrimination Test (1958), the Goldman-Fristoe Test of Articulation (1969), and the Peabody Picture Vocabulary Test (PPVT)(Dunn & Dunn, 1965). With regard to the expressive portion of the NSST, for example, the authors demonstrated numerous examples of nonstandard English responses to standard English stimuli which would be considered to be incorrect given the scoring parameters of the test. Among these examples are the use of pronominal apposition and the omission of third person singular present tense markers as illustrated in the response "The baby, he sleeping" to the stimulus "The baby is sleeping." On the Wepman, confusion may be created by interdialectal homophony, or the tendency for two words that are different in one dialect to be perceived as the same in another dialect. Thus, the Black English speaker's response to the presentation of the work pairs "clothe-clove" and "sheaf-sheath" is likely to be that the words are the same, a response which would be regarded as erroneous given the test's interpretative guidelines. Common dialectal variations which may be produced by children during the administration of the Goldman-Fristoe and considered to be misarticulations are deletion of the word-final nasal consonant, the substitution of /t/ for the voiceless "th" sound, and the devoicing of the /d/ in word-final position as might occur during the productions of "gun," "thumb," and "bed." Sources of difficulty for the Black English speaker, among others, on the PPVT are stimuli for which the subject uses a different word ("engineer," "cobbler"), or which the child pronounces differently ("finger," "ambulance"), or which the child uses in a manner different from the test ("hook").

Related research reinforces the concerns of Wolfram, Williams, and Taylor about the biases of speech-language diagnostic procedures and underscores the need to be vigilant in the interpretation of test results. Bliss and Allen (1981) investigated the extent to which black preschool children responded in Black English and standard English on the expressive items of the NSST, as well as the Fluharty Preschool Screening Test (1974) and the Test of Grammatical Structure (Bliss & Allen, 1976). Prior to the administration of the tests, the examiners were trained to identify the phonological, syntactic-semantic, and communication styles of Black English speakers. The results from all three tests indicated that the subjects used both dialectal and standard English features, but that the younger subjects, who were between two-and-a-half and three years of age, produced twice as many dialectal variations as older subjects. The significance of these results is that speech-language clinicians need to be particularly circumspect in their assessments of young black children who may still be functioning at a prebidialectal stage of devel-

opment and using linguistic characteristics which could be miscon-
strued as being pathologically varient. In a study which focused
solely upon the Fluharty, Bountress and Hayes (1983) selected
ninety-three four-and-five-year-old black kindergarten children who
were from lower socioeconomic-level families and sixty-five white
middle-class children as subjects. The Fluharty was administered
and an item analysis utilized to determine which items, apart from
those designated by the test authors as dialectal variations, were
most frequently indicated as being incorrect. Four items were found
to significantly differentiate black subjects from white subjects, with
black subjects making from two to four times as many errors on the
items as white subjects. These items included the omission of plural
markers and the omission of forms of "have" which have been commonly described as being characteristic of Black English. In another
study, Duchan and Baskervill (1977) directed their concerns to the
Grammatic Closure Subtest of the Illinois Test of Psycholinguistic
Abilities (ITPA) (Kirk, McCarthy, & Kirk, 1968), a measure on
which black children have a reported tendency to perform poorly.
The subtest was administered to seventy normal black and white elementary school children, with twenty-seven items that measured
morphologic inflections being analyzed. The results indicated that
black and white subjects differed in their responses to one-third of
the items presented, suggesting that the likely reason for black children's reportedly poor performance on the subtest may be because of
culturally-related linguistic differences.

While there is a great need for more studies such as the preceding
which examine the racially- and culturally-based linguistic biases of
commonly administered speech and language tests, there is an
equally urgent need to develop new approaches for diagnosing
speech and language disorders in an unbiased manner. Evard and
Sabers (1979) have suggested that three such possible approaches
are to develop new tests, modify existing tests, and develop local test
norms. The first approach has been demonstrated through the development of tests such as the Test for Auditory Comprehension of
Language: English/Spanish (Carrow, 1973) and The Mexican-
American Inventory of Receptive Abilities (Nelson-Burgess & Meyerson, 1975) which were developed for Mexican-American children,
the Denver Articulation Screening Exam (Drumwright et al, 1973)
which was developed for a broader cross-section of non-standard

English speakers, and the Screening Kit of Language Development (Bliss & Allen, 1983) which contains normative data for speakers of Black English. However, as Evard and Sabers indicate, not only is the development of tests costly and time-consuming, it is likely to culminate in a tool which has only limited utility beyond the geographical locale and population on which it was normed. The second approach entails the modification of an existing test's items or responses so that they are reflective of the cultural and linguistic backgrounds of the population to which the test is administered. Apart from problems related to cross-cultural translation, the major drawback of this procedure is that the test is rendered invalid because the modified responses are no longer representative of the normative data obtained from the test's original standardization sample. The third approach discussed by Evard and Sabers is the development of local norms for specific tests while maintaining standardized procedures. For example, the authors cite projects in which the Templin-Darley Tests of Articulation (1969) and subtests of the ITPA were normed on specific ethnic-racial groups such as blacks and Mexican-Americans. Such a procedure, while more cost-effective than the other options, is still limited in its ability to be generalized to similar populations in other locales, a limitation which is also common to the vast majority of speech-language tests presently being used. As Evard and Sabers conclude, because there are no simple solutions to the problem of constructing speech and language tests and procedures for use with diverse ethnic and racial groups, clinicians must select which of the three procedures is most appropriate in a given situation.

Regardless of the specific diagnostic tests used in the assessment of the speech and language abilities of minority groups, a fundamental competency which clinicians must possess is a knowledge of dialectal variations. In particular, clinicians must be acutely aware of the local variations which are used in their geographical area and, according to Labov (1975), the degree to which such variations are entrenched. Such knowledge allows the clinician to observe the similarity between local children's dialectal variations and those commonly-occurring characteristics which have been described in national studies. This is of importance because it provides the clinician with first-hand evidence of the consistency of non-standard English. However, knowledge of local norms also allows for the recognition of local linguistic characteristics which vary from both nationally-recognized dialectal characteristics as well as standard English. A carefully compiled corpus of local variations will aid the clinician in determining if, for example, a black child is using pathological variations from both standard English and Black English or if he is using characteristics which, while differing from both standard and Black English, are common to his immediate linguistic community. Information of this nature must be clearly understood by the clinician so that he can recognize the linguistically biased items in diagnostic tests and so that he can discount such items when making accurate diagnostic decisions. Labov (1975) and Adler (1979) have suggested a number of procedures for obtaining information about local dialectal variations, such as spontaneous speech sampling, classroom observation, observation outside of the classroom, carefully structured face-to-face interviews in which the subject and a peer are allowed to interact verbally, and group discussion sessions in which group composition is determined by the subjects. However, the most commonly employed and useful method is the sentence repetition task in which subjects are asked to listen to and repeat sentences presented orally by the examiner. Complete repetitions, omissions, and revisions of linguistic units are analyzed and can be compared within and between linguistic communities for the purpose of developing a corpus of regional variations. Labov and Adler recommend that such tasks include the use of sentences which contain both standard and non-standard rules, while Hemingway, Montague, and Bradley (1981) and Bountress and Rochelle (1982) have constructed tests which are limited to standard English stimuli. The initial results obtained from both procedures suggest that such activities are of considerable value in assessing bidialectal facility and in compiling information about local linguistic variations.

Teaching Standard English

As is the case with diagnostic procedures, the teaching of standard English to dialect speakers requires that the speech-language clinician not only modify his traditional perspective but also his traditional approaches to clinical intervention and professional interaction with teachers and parents. The teaching model itself, represents a radical departure from the clinician's traditional role, not only because there are no "therapy" procedures as such, but because the rationale for intervention is different. As the programs described by Seymour and Seymour (1977), Adler (1979), and Feigenbaum (1975) have illustrated, the language pathology model uses standard English as the goal while the language difference, or bidialectal, model focuses upon the appropriate use of both standard and nonstandard English. Therefore, children who use linguistic variations that differ from national and local norms for standard and nonstandard English would be appropriate candidates for therapy, while those whose language differs from standard English but conforms to national and local non-standard English norms would be candidates for programs using the bidialectal model. Because of the frequent confusion which occurs regarding the purpose of using the bidialectal model, the preceding discussion deserves reiteration. The goal of bidialectal programs is to have the speaker learn standard English so that he can use it in situations where it is appropriate and beneficial to him while encouraging him to use the native dialect when it is, likewise, appropriate and beneficial.

The procedures used in many bidialectal programs, such as those described by Feigenbaum (1975), Adler (1979), and Johnson (1971), have two principal features: recognition of and respect for the legitimacy of the native dialect and the use of techniques which compare and contrast features of the native and standard dialects. As has been discussed previously, most speech-language clinicians should have at least a fundamental awareness of the legitimacy of social dialects. However, it is basic to the administration of bidialectal programs that the clinician convey that awareness to the student. Therefore, at the initiation of intervention programs, the clinician must create an atmosphere in which the student will feel free to interact because he understands that his utterances are valued. While attention is focused upon the differences and similarities between the child's "home" language and the "school" language, the child's dialect is never criticized. The legitimacy and value of the native dialect are emphasized as well as the realities of language discrimination and the social, educational, and economic advantages of using standard English. It is of particular importance that, at the outset of the program, the child be encouraged to continue to use his dialect with peers and also to become cognizant of the need for standard English use in settings such as the classroom.

The teaching methodology, itself, is based upon principles of pedagogy which are commonly used in the teaching of foreign languages and, according to Feigenbaum (1975), relies upon the assumption that it is easier for the student to comprehend the systematic differences between non-standard and standard if he understands the regularity of his own language. Therefore, teaching drills focus upon the comparing and contrasting of the native dialect with standard English. The lessons are developed after the discussions between teacher and student of the legitimacy of non-standard dialects and after a thorough assessment of the student's language. This assessment should identify those dialectal features which are particularly resistant to dialectal shift and which create communicative problems for the speaker in settings where the use of standard English is appropriate. These features, both phonological and grammatical, then become the targets for contrastive and comparative analysis. While there are numerous ways to organize such lessons, the format described by Feigenbaum has potential applicability to a variety of clinical settings. The graduated steps which comprise this approach are presentation, discrimination drills, identification drills, translation drills, and response drills. The presentation activity is a very brief exercise in which two sentences, one standard and one non-standard, are presented and the student is asked to describe how they differ. The purpose of this activity is to have the student differentiate standard from non-standard English without the necessity of a complex grammatical explanation. In discrimination drills, the student is orally presented stimulus word or sentence pairs which are combinations of standard and/or non-standard stimuli ("masks-masks"; "masks-masses") and the student must indicate if the paired stimuli are the same or different. Identification drills require the student to identify a single word or sentence as being standard or non-standard English. In translation drills, the student must translate a word or sentence from standard ("He works hard") to non-standard ("He work hard") and from non-standard to standard. Feigenbaum notes that these exercises are of additional value because they provide opportunities for students to hear the standard forms which they will eventually be required to produce. The response drills are less rigid than the previous grammatical manipulation activities and allow the student the opportunity of speaking in a more natural conversational manner. The teacher presents specific cuing behaviors in an attempt to elicit specific grammatical responses. For example, the teacher may present "We waited here," and the child repeats the stimulus. The teacher then presents "They" and the student uses that word in the sentence context, giving "They waited here." The teacher might then produce "I" with the student expected to produce "I waited here." The exercises may be graduated in complexity so that cuing may eventually elicit a broad range of responses with increasing responsibility for the generation and production of linguistic features being assigned to the student.

Such approaches as Feigenbaum's and the similar programs of Adler and Johnson warrant attention from the speech-language clinician who works with dialect speakers. However, it would be short-sighted to assume that the entire scope of intervention is limited to direct teaching activities with the student. As with the speech-language disordered child, a full program of intervention requires interaction with both teachers and parents, but, as was the case in the clinician's role as a teacher of bidialectalism, these activities require some variation from traditional role functions. For example, interaction with the classroom teacher should focus upon service as a resource consultant, a role which may include advocacy and the transmission of information as well as the structuring of developmental language programs. Adler (1979; 1980) and Baskervill (1977) emphasize that the clinician has an important function in dispelling prejudicial attitudes by presenting teacher in-services that describe dialectal variations, the relationship of language and intelligence, the biases of standardized tests, and current research trends. While public school clinicians cannot provide direct services to dialect speakers because of the legal definition of their professional duties, they can help teachers to structure appropriate programs. The range of such activities includes the eliminating of cultural biases in language-oriented classroom materials, differentiating between dialects and pathological variations, and developing programs which will increase verbalization in minority children. Of additional importance is helping the classroom teacher to instill positive attitudes in children regarding their dialects through the teaching of linguistic origins and the similarities which exist between non-standard and standard dialects, as well as through the demonstration of genuine respect for the children's language.

The importance of the speech-language clinician's interaction with the parents of dialect speakers is that such activity promotes the transfer of information which is learned in bidialectal programs through parental monitoring of home assignments and the providing of reinforcement for attempts at style shifting. As is the case with children who have speech and language disorders, maximal progress cannot be made without a motivated and knowledgeable parent. To ensure that parents will become an integral part of the intervention program, the clinician needs to stimulate ongoing parental participation, gauge parental sensitivity to and understanding of pertinent issues, and clarify these issues through well-considered instruction. Information regarding participation by lower socioeconomic level minority populations in speech-language programs is scarce, with the few studies that have been done indicating limited participation (Screen & Taylor, 1972; Bountress, Jones, and Mayfield, 1983). However, when the issue has been related to the effect of language differences on educational placement, as in the Ann Arbor decision, minority parents have responded with highly effective activism. In any event, the clinician should anticipate potential barriers to full parental involvement by becoming aware of problems imposed by economic and transportation factors as well as by suspicion and lack of information regarding middle-class agencies. Specifically, the clinician should consider the efficacy of home visitations, develop better channels of communication, and identify sources of financial support for families wishing to avail themselves of clinical services. Parent instructional activities should focus upon the imparting of background information on dialects as well as specific transfer activities. For example, Adler (1980) suggests that the parents should be instructed regarding the influence of language differences upon children's educational success, the nature of bidialectalism, and the legitimacy of dialectal variations, and should also be provided with periodic in-service instruction to facilitate the development and transfer of activities which parallel those used by the clinician. It is such activities which, when coordinated with the clinician and classroom teacher's instruction, considerably enhance the child's development of bidialectalism and adjustment to the school environment.

WHEN SHOULD DIALECTAL INTERVENTION PROGRAMS BE INITIATED?

The appropriate time to initiate dialectal intervention programs, and, specifically, the facilitation of bidialectalism, is not clear. There has been considerable discussion regarding the topic, with two discernible tendencies emerging. Some researchers and educators claim that instruction in standard English should begin in the early elementary school years and, in some cases, kindergarten and preschool, while others strongly advocate the postponing of second dialect instruction until the secondary school level. The latter argument has been discussed in varying degrees of detail by Labov (1964; 1975), Wolfram and Shuy (1974), Burling (1973), and Johnson (1971), among others, who state that dialect speakers should be taught standard English when they are sufficiently aware of the need for it. Because, as Labov (1964) noted, children's awareness of the social consequences related to language usage does not correspond to adult perceptions until the ages of fourteen or fifteen years, their self-perceived need for linguistic change is not urgent. Furthermore, students may not be satisfactorily motivated to learn standard English until they enter junior high school or high school and become more conscious of the role of language in their proposed educational or professional careers. These researchers have also stated that, contrary to the arguments of many educators, it is not necessary to teach standard English to dialect speakers before they have been taught reading and writing skills because there is no linguistic evidence to support the contention that reading and writing problems result from the use of dialect. Finally, there are proponents of this position who feel that the principal purpose of the elementary school should be to emphasize the teaching of reading and not the instruction of standard English.

Advocates of early intervention, including a number of speech-language clinicians, argue that the purpose of developing bidialectal programs is to provide the child with a less-stigmatized means of expressing himself which can serve as a tool for competing in the middle-class milieu. If such programs are postponed, the child is deprived of that tool and exposed to the negative and potentially harmful attitudes that are frequently directed at dialect speakers. It has been suggested that while bidialectalism may be only a stop-gap measure against linguistic and cultural bias, it must suffice until the attitudes of educators and employers are changed. Advocates of this position have also pointed out that the preschool years represent an important period of linguistic growth in which the child demonstrates remarkable facility in the development of lexical, phonological, and syntactic abilities as illustrated by the relative ease with which foreign languages are learned. Substantiation of this point with regard to dialect speakers is found in the results of bidialectal programs described by Adler (1979). The programs developed were based upon principles of bidialectal teaching which have been set forth by Johnson (1971) and Feigenbaum (1975) and administered to one group of four- and five-year-old Head Start children and to another group of children enrolled in kindergarten through third grade in rural Tennessee. The results obtained from both programs indicated increases in both the quantity and quality of linguistic production as well as in participatory behaviors. A final argument presented by supporters of the early-intervention position is that young children's awareness of the contextual appropriateness of language may develop earlier than is frequently assumed. For example, Bliss and Allen (1981) found that black preschool children between the ages of two-and-a-half and four years demonstrated a knowledge of both black and standard English in three test situations, and Geiger and Greenberg (1976) found that ten-year-old black children were able to discriminate dialectal differences from standard English forms on the basis of syntactic distinctions.

Another possible rationale which may be of value in supporting the argument for early intervention is based upon research which has examined stages in the acquistion of standard English. Labov (1964) has delineated six such stages: a needs-oriented basic grammar, a peer-oriented vernacular, and adult-influenced stage developed concomitantly with increased social perception, stylistic variation characterized by modification toward the prestige dialect, consistent use of standard, and a full-range repertoire for a variety of occasions. Factors which may influence a speaker's speed and manner of transition through such stages are the relationship of the speaker to the prestige group, exposure to standard English, group reference, social context, peer pressure and consequences meted out by teachers for using nonstandard characteristics. The likely conclusion which could be drawn from an analysis of these varied factors is that the age at which the child makes the most significant transition from the non-standard to the standard dialect is highly variable. However, a number of developmental studies which focused upon lower socioeconomic level black children's acquisition of standard English not only suggest that this period of transition may be fairly uniform but that it generally occurs well before the junior high school years. For example, the research of Ramer and Rees (1973) indicates that the period of greatest decline in use of dialect features for five of six standard English constructions studied occurred between preschool and fifth grade, and three of these between preschool and first grade. However, because no population between first grade and fifth grade was examined, it is impossible to conclude how much before fifth grade the period of greatest decline for some of the dialect features occurred. A series of studies by Bountress has suggested that this period may be closer to first grade than to fifth grade. In an investigation of six standard English constructions, Bountress (1977) found that there was a large and uniform decline of dialectal variations in the language of seven-year-old black children from Texas. A related study (Bountress, 1978) of black English speaker's comprehension of pronoun reference indicated mastery at approximately the same age. A later study which focused upon the development of a dialect screening test for establishing local norms in Virginia (Bountress & Rochelle, 1982), as well as a recent follow-up study, also suggested significant declines in dialect use between the ages of six and eight years. While conclusions based upon this information must be considered to be speculative at this time, these studies suggest the presence of a period during the early primary years when there is a significant decline in dialect use. The identificication of such a period is of clinical value for not only the establishment of reference points in the charting of typical and atypical patterns of standard English acquisition, but also in selecting opportune times for more easily facilitating the teaching of standard English to dialect speakers.

While most speech-language clinicians have been trained to appreciate the value of early intervention, it may be that, in some settings, or with some populations, it is not feasible to begin the actual process of teaching standard English through contrastive analysis in, or before, the early primary grades. In such cases or preparatory to the programs of Feigenbaum and others, the clinician may, as Geiger and Greenberg (1976) suggest, want to initiate instruction by focusing only on paralinguistic or lexical features. Another alternative is presented by Loban (1968) who recommended that the preschool and kindergarten years should be for the adjustment of the child and the constructing of an accepting environment by the teacher. The primary grades should emphasize the practicing of standard English phonemes through participation in plays and skits, the modeling of a variety of dialects and learning to respect dialectal origins, and engaging in informal contrastive language exercises. In grades four, five, and six, students should participate in discussions in which contemporary dialects are discussed, in plays which utilize a variety of dialects, and in exercises where sentences are read which contain dialectal variations with students being required to decide which are standard or nonstandard. Loban states that grades five, six, and seven are suitable for discussions concerning the social, educational, and employment consequences of nonstandard language. While Logan's program may not provide sufficient didactic structure for some clinicians, it represents a compromise between programs which advocate intervention at the preschool and early primary levels and those that advocate intervention at the junior high and high school levels.

There is no easy resolution to the question of when dialectal programs should be initiated, but perhaps it is in the best interests of the student that the speech-language clinician draw from the varied perspectives which exist. While early intervention would appear to be the most reasonable choice, the clinician must make this decision only with the ongoing input of parents and other professionals and based upon a realistic assessment of the educational and occupational goals and social, cultural and psychological needs of the student.

REFERENCES

Adler, S. Dialectal Differences: Professional and Clinical Implications. *Journal of Speech and Hearing Disorders*, 1971, 36, 90-100.

Adler, S. *Poverty Children and Their Language.* New York: Grune & Stratton, 1979.

Adler, S. The Pediatric Language Specialist: An Innovative Approach to Early Language Intervention and the Role of the Speech-language Clinician. *Speech and Language: Advances in Basic Research and Practice*, 1980, 3, 99-127.

American Speech-Language-Hearing Association position paper on social dialects. *Asha*, 1983, 25, 23-24.

Ammons, R., & Ammons, C. The Full-range Picture Vocabulary Test. Missoula, Montana: Psychological Test Specialists, 1958.

Andersland, P. Maternal and Environmental Factors Related to Success in

Speech Improvement Training. *Journal of Speech and Hearing Research*, 1961, 4, 79-90.

Baratz, J. Who Should Do What to Whom and Why? *Florida Foreign Language Reporter*, 1969, 7, 75-77.

Baskervill, R. The Speech-language Pathologist: A Resource Consultant for Enhancing Standard English English Competencies Among Inner-city Children. *Language, Speech, and Hearing Services in Schools*, 1977, 8, 245-249.

Bernstein, B. A Sociolinguistic Approach to Language Learning. In J. Gould (Ed.), *Penguin Survey of the Social Sciences*. Baltimore: Penguin, 1965.

Bernstein, B. A Sociolinguistic Approach to Socialization: With Some Reference to Educability. In F. Williams (Ed.), *Language and Poverty*. Chicago: Markham Publishing Company, 1970.

Blank, M. & Solomon, F. How Shall the Disadvantaged Child Be Taught? *Child Development*, 1969, 40, 47-61.

Bliss, L., & Allen, D. Black English Responses on Selected Language Tests. *Journal of Communication Disorders*, 1981, 14, 225-233.

Bliss, L., & Allen, D. Test of Grammatical Structure. Unpublished, 1976.

Bliss, L., & Allen, D. The Screening Kit of Language Development. Baltimore: University Park Press, 1983.

Bountress, N. Approximations of Selected Standard English Sentences by Speakers of Black English *Journal of Speech and Hearing Research*, 1977, 20, 254-262.

Bountress, N. Attitudes and Training of Public School Clinicians Providing Services to Speakers of Black English. *Language, Speech, and Hearing Services in Schools*, 1980a, 11, 41-49.

Bountress, N. Comprehension of Pronominal Reference by Speakers of Black English. *Journal of Speech and Hearing Research*, 1978, 21, 96-102.

Bountress, N. The Ann Arbor Decision: Implications for the Speech-language Pathologist. *Asha*, 1980b, 22, 543-544.

Bountress, N., & Bountress, M. The Influence of Racial Experimenter Effects on Mean Length of Utterance. Paper presented at the annual convention of the American Speech-Language-Hearing Association, Toronto, 1982.

Bountress, N., & Hayes, J. An Examination of Linguistic Bias on the Fluharty Screening Test. Paper presented at the annual convention of the American Speech-Language-Hearing Association, Toronto, 1982.

Bountress, N., & Jones, R., & Mayfield, R. Attitudes of Parents of Black Communicatively Disordered Children. Paper presented at the annual convention of the American Speech-Language-Hearing Association, Cincinnati, 1983.

Bountress, N., & Rochelle, M. Initial Results from an Elicited Imitation Black Dialect Screening Test. Paper presented at the annual convention of the American Speech-Language-Hearing Association, Toronto, 1982.

Bronstein, A. Sociolinguistics and the Speech and Language Pathologist. *Asha*, 1973, 15, 694-697.

Burling, R. Talking to Teachers About Social Dialects. *Language Learning*, 1971, 21, 221-234.

Caplan, S., & Ruble, R. A Study of Culturally Imposed Factors on School Achievement in a Metropolitan Area. *Journal of Educational Research,* 1964, 58, 16-21.

Carrow, E. Test for Auditory Comprehension of Language. Austin: *Learning Concepts,* 1973.

Carson, A., & Rabin, A. Verbal Comprehension and Communication in Negro and White Children. *Journal of Educational Psychology,* 1960, 51, 47-51.

Chomsky, N. Current Issues in Linguistic Theory. In J. Fodor S J. Katz (Ed.), *The Structure of Language.* Englewood Cliffs, New Jersey: Prentice-Hall, 1964.

Clark, A., & Richards, C. Auditory Discrimination Among Economically Disadvantaged and Non-disadvantaged Preschool Children. *Exceptional Children,* 1966, 33, 259-266.

Cohn, W. On the Language of Lower-class Children. *The School Review,* 1959, 67, 435-440.

Deutsch, C. Auditory Discrimination and Learning. *Merrill-Palmer Quarterly,* 1964, 10, 277-296.

Deutsch, M. The Role of Social Class in Language Development and Cognition. *American Journal of Orthopsychiatry,* 1965, 35, 78-88.

Drumwright, A., Van Natta, P., Camp, B., & Frankenburg, W. The Denver Articulation Screening Examination. *Journal of Speech and Hearing Disorders,* 1973, 38, 3-14.

Duchan, J., & Baskervill, R. Responses of Black and White Children on the Grammatic Closure Subtest of the ITPA. *Language, Speech, and Hearing Services in Schools,* 1977, 8, 126-132.

Dunn, L. Special Education for the Mentally Retarded: Is Much of it Justifiable? *Exceptional Children,* 1968, 35, 5-22.

Dunn, L., & Dunn, L. Peabody Picture Vocabulary Test. Nashville: American Guidance Service, 1959.

Education of Handicapped Children: Implementation of the Education of the Handicapped Act. *Federal Register,* 1977, 42, 42474-42518.

Eisenson, J., & Ogilvie, M. *Communicative Disorders in Children.* New York: Macmillan Publishing Company, 1983.

Evard, B., & Sabers, D. Speech and Language Testing With Distinct Ethnicracial Groups: A Survey of Procedures for Improving Validity. *Journal of Speech and Hearing Disorders,* 1979, 44, 271-281.

Fasold, R., & Wolfram, W. Some Linguistic Features of Negro Dialect. *Language, Speech and Hearing Services in Schools,* 1972, 3, 16-49.

Feigenbaum, I. The Use of Non-standard English in Teaching Standard: Contrast and Comparison. In P. Stoller (Ed.), *Black American English.* New York: Dell Publishing Company, 1975.

Fluharty, N. The Design and Standardization of a Speech and Language Screening Test for Use with Preschool Children. *Journal of Speech and Hearing Disorders,* 1974, 39, 75-88.

Frentz, T. Children's Comprehension of Standard and Negro Non-standard English Sentences. *Speech Monographs,* 1971, 38, 10-16.

Geiger, S., & Greenberg, B. The Black Child's Ability to Discriminate Dialect

Differences: Implications for Dialect Language Programs. *Language, Speech, and Hearing Services in Schools,* 1976, 7, 28-32.

Goldman, R., & Fristoe, M. *Test of Articulation.* Circle Pines, Minnesota: American Guidance Service, 1969.

Hechinger, F. Suit Brings Changes in Special Education. *New York Times,* November 1979.

Hemingway, B., Montague, J., & Bradley, R. Preliminary Data on Revision of a Sentence Repetition Test for Language Screening with Black First Grade Children. *Language, Speech, and Hearing Services in Schools,* 1981, 12, 153-159.

Hess, R., & Shipman, V. Early Experience and the Socialization of Cognitive Modes of Children. *Child Development,* 1965, 36, 869-886.

Irwin, O. Infant Speech: The Effect of Family Occupational Status and of Age on Use of Sound Types. *Journal of Speech and Hearing Disorders,* 1948, 13, 224-226.

Jensen, A. How Much Can We Boost IQ and Scholastic Achievement? *Harvard Educational Review,* 1969, 39, 1-123.

John, V. The Intellectual Development of Slum Children. *American Journal of Orthopsychiatry,* 1963, 33, 813-822.

Johnson, K. R. Should Black Children Learn Standard English? In M. Imhoof (Ed.), *Social and Educational Insights into Teaching Standard English to Speakers of Other Dialects.* Bloomington, Indiana: Indiana University Press, 1971.

Kirk, S., McCarthy, J., & Kirk, W. Illinois Test of Psycholinguistic Abilities. Urbana, Illinois: University of Illinois Press, 1968.

Labov Explores Significance of Black English Court Case. *English Journal,* 1981, 70, 75-76.

Labov, W. Stages in the Acquistion of Standard English. In R. Shuy (Ed.), *Social Dialects and Language Learning.* Champaign, Illinois: National Council of Teachers of English, 1964.

Labov, W. *The Study of Non-standard English.* Urbana, Illinois: National Council of Teachers of English, 1975.

Labov, W. The Logic of Non-standard English. In F. Williams (Ed.), *Language and Poverty.* Chicago: Markham Publishing Company, 1970.

Lawton, D. Social Class Language Differences in Group Discussions. *Language and Speech,* 1964, 7, 183-204.

Lee, L. Northwestern Syntax Screening Test. Evanston, Illinois: Northwestern University Press, 1971.

Linguistic Society of America Statement and Resolution on Language and Intelligence. *Linguistic Society of America Bulletin,* March 1972, 17-22.

Loban, W. Teaching Children Who Speak Social Class Dialects. *Elementary English,* 1968, 45, 592-599.

Martin Luther King Junior Elementary School Children v. Ann Arbor school district. *F. Supp.,* 1979, 473, 1371-1391.

McDavid, R. On a Hierarchy of Values: The Children of the Dialectologist. In J. Akin et al (Ed.), *Language Behavior.* The Hague: Mouton Press, 1970.

Mercer, J. *Labeling the Mentally Retarded.* Berkeley: University of California Press, 1973.

Nelson-Burgess, S., & Meyerson, J. MIRA: A Concept in Receptive Language

Assessment of Bilingual Children. *Language, Speech, and Hearing Services in Schools*, 1975, 6, 24-28.

Ramer, A., & Rees, N. Selected Aspects of the Development of English Morphology in Black American Children of Low Socioeconomic Background. *Journal of Speech and Hearing Research*, 1973, 4, 569-576.

Ramsey, I. A Comparison of First Grade Negro Dialect Speakers' Comprehension of Standard English and Negro Dialect. *Elementary English*, 1972, 49, 688-696.

Raph, J. Language and Speech Deficits in Culturally Disadvantaged Children. *Journal of Speech and Hearing Disorders*, 1967, 32, 203-214.

Screen, R., & Taylor, H. Relevancy of Speech and Hearing Facilities to the Black Community. *Language, Speech, and Hearing Services in Schools*, 1972, 3, 56-61.

Seymour, H., & Seymour, C. A Therapeutic Model for Communicative Disorders Among Children Who Speak Black English Vernacular. *Journal of Speech and Hearing Disorders*, 1977, 42, 247-256.

Shuy, R. Sociolinguistic Strategies for Studying Urban Speech. In M. Imhoof (Ed.), *Social and Educational Insights into Teaching Standard English to Speakers of Other Dialects*. Bloomington, Indiana: Indiana University Press, 1971.

Stewart, W. Non-standard Speech and the Teaching of English. Washington, D.C.: Center for Applied Linguistics, 1964.

Taylor, O. Communication Disorders in Blacks. In B. Williams & O. Taylor (Ed.), *International Conference on Black Communication*. New York: Rockefeller Foundation, 1980.

Templin, M. *Certain Language Skills in Children*. Minneapolis: University of Minnesota Press, 1957.

Templin, M., & Darley, F. The Templin-Darley Tests of Articulation. Iowa City: University of Iowa, 1969.

Terrell, S., & Terrell, F. Effects of Speaking Black English upon Employment Opportunities. *Asha*, 1983, 25, 27-34.

Wepman, J. Auditory Discrimination Test. Chicago: Language Research Associates, 1958.

Williams, F. Some Preliminaries and Prospects. In F. Williams (Ed.), *Language and Poverty*. Chicago: Markham Publishing Company, 1970.

Williams, F. Training and Retraining of Speech, Hearing, and Language School Specialists. *Language, Speech, and Hearing Services in Schools*, 1972, 3, 50-55.

Wolfram, W. Detroit Negro Speech. Washington, D.C.: Center for Applied Linguistics, 1969.

Wolfram, W. Speech Pathology and Dialect Differences. Arlington, Virginia: Center for Applied Linguistics, 1979.

Wolfram, W., & Fasold, R. *Social Dialects in American English*. Englewood Cliffs, New Jersey: Prentice-Hall, 1974.

Wolfram, W., Williams, R., & Taylor, O. Dialectal Bias of Language Assessment Instruments. Paper presented at the annual convention of the American Speech and Hearing Association, San Francisco, 1972.

Chapter V

THE PEDIATRIC LANGUAGE SPECIALIST:

An Innovative Approach to Early Language Intervention and the Role of the Speech-Language Clinician*

SOL ADLER and IOWANA A. WHITMAN TIMS

I. INTRODUCTION

DURING the beginning years of the development of the profession of speech pathology, our professional concerns were almost entirely focused on the client possessing speech and/or voice impairments. During and following World War II, a sudden escalation of interest occurred regarding the problems of the hard-of-hearing client. In the early 1960s, we expanded our job description to include the diverse language problems of exceptional children. The late 1960s witnessed a further expansion into the linguistic differences of culturally different and poor children.

Today we are much involved with the verbal and nonverbal communication skills manifested by children, no matter how different or disabling their condition. This concern and involvement have

---

*As presented in Speech and Language: *Advances in Basic Research and Practice,* Volume 3, 1980

created a need for (1) professional workers knowledgeable about language development, disorders, and differences in children; and (2) innovative programs for such children. However, in part due to the inappropriate or ineffective teaching and treating programs designed for such children (or to the lack of any program for such children), Public Law 94-142 was mandated; this law demands that our society provide an appropriate education for all children. However, before we can provide such an education to these children, it should be acknowledged that we must first give them the necessary language tools-the touchstone upon which their academic skills must ultimately rest.

As our job description is expanded, so must academic courses and practica, as well as American Speech-Language-Hearing Association (ASHA) requirements, be expanded to meet the growing clinical demands placed upon the speech and hearing specialist. Unfortunately, such expansion is slow in coming. For example, in the late 1970s, we altered our title so that we are now recognized as speech-language and hearing clinicians; but the courses, practica, and ASHA requirements have not changed sufficiently to parallel this alteration in our title. Nor have our philosophies or clinical strategies been altered in any significant way. Most academic training programs continue to produce "parochial" clinicians; that is, clinicians who have been taught to use orthodox or conventional clinical programming in their various interactions with language-defective or, more to the point, language-different children.

The quantity or number of early-childhood or pediatric language specialists available to cater in unorthodox ways to language-deficient or -different children is, in fact, limited; the quality or level of training of these available workers is also severely limited. There are simply too few of our professional peers available who possess extensive training in pediatric language — its development, disorders, and differences.

There are a variety of educational and treatment concepts with which pediatric language specialists should be familiar and be able to translate into effective programming. For example, (1) intensive family participation involving (a) counseling programs, (b) education programs, and — as is relevant — (c) parent-infant stimulation programs; (2) nonverbal communication systems for neuromuscularly impaired or mentally retarded children; (3) outreach programming to rural and inner-city poor; (4) appropriate testing methodologies and the reporting of reliable and valid data, particularly as these data relate to poor children; (5) innovative and appropriate teaching of developmental language as well as the treatment of language deficiencies in early language intervention programs such as day-care and head-start. This would include the ability to distinguish between deficiencies and differences in the paralinguistic and linguistic utterances of culturally different children, and the ability to utilize a bidialectal and bicultural teaching strategy in the teaching-treating program.

It is not the intent of this chapter to explore in depth all of the concepts previously noted, but rather to discuss in some detail the last-named topic: early intervention strategies with the culturally different and poor child.

The Pediatric Language Programs at the University of Tennessee

In the past two decades, many millions of government dollars have been spent to increase the number of day-care and head-start centers throughout the country; unfortunately, little has been done to enhance the effectiveness of these programs with respect to the communication-skill development of the children enrolled. At the University of Tennessee, two programs, the Pediatric Language Institute and the Language Laboratory, have been addressing this problem. In the former program we train day-care workers — both professionals and paraprofessionals in a 13-county area in East Tennessee — to become aware of the dynamics in volved in language acquisition: their biopsycho- and sociolinguistic dynamics, and how best to teach developmental language skills to these children through both formalized and incidental language learning strategies. In the latter program, we maintain two day-care centers on our campus to develop a model early language intervention program for children possessing mild to moderate language deficiencies. In this program, we have both taught and treated linguistic differences and deficiencies.* In another program, the Pediatric Language Clinic, we provide (1) infant stimulation training, and (2) counseling (affective, financial, and educational), to rural poor families with exceptional and language-retarded children.

---

*These concepts are enunciated in more detail in the senior author's book, *Poverty Children and Their Language: Implications for Teaching and Treating*. New York: Grune & Stratton, 1979.

II. JOB DESCRIPTION OF THE PEDIATRIC LANGUAGE
SPECIALIST

We have expressed the idea of expanding the professional role of the clinician, particularly in his or her affiliation with certain early childhood education programs. Part of our concern is with the limitations associated with the job role that traditionally has been assumed by the clinician in his or her contact with preschool children and the ultimate effects upon the children enrolled in the programs. The clinician usually has functioned in the capacity of an itinerant worker who provides diagnostic and treatment services to children with defective speech or language patterns. One of the limitations of the job role is that many preschool children do not receive appropriate assistance with their communicative needs. They are taught developmental language skills using only standard English as the mode of instruction. All too frequently, the poor child's dialectal speech patterns are considered substandard and are treated as errors to be corrected. However, more recently, and perhaps in reaction to the previously noted criticisms, many dialectal speech patterns of poor children are being regarded as acceptable utterances, not to be altered. Representative of this approach is the ruling by U.S. District Judge Charles Joiner that the Ann Arbor school district in Michigan "take steps to help its teachers to recognize the home language of the student" (Associated Press release).

The fallacy of these unicultural-unidialectal approaches to treating developmental language is well recognized. But the current job description of most clinicians is, in fact, related to a unicultural underpinning. It is this philosophical stance that is most in need of alteration. Any treatment program that uses standard English as the only acceptable instructional mode and requires the child to abandon his or her dialect and speak only standard English ignores current sociolinguistic data which attest to the legitimacy of many cultural dialects (Labov, 1966; Dillard, 1972). More importantly, this type of approach may lead to confusion and despair, and may be detrimental to the self-concept that is fostered by the child whose cultural dialect (the language spoken by his parents, siblings, peers, etc.) is criticized and possibly eradicated by the remediation program that is used. But, similarly, any education program that accepts the dialectal patterns without attempting to teach the child to

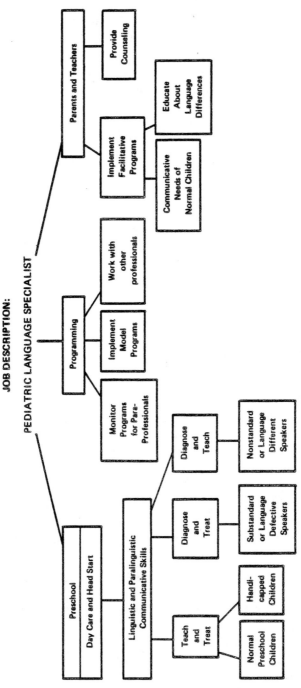

Figure 5-1. Diagram of professional skills that the pediatric language specialist should possess in order to teach and treat communicative skills to preschool children effectively.

be diglossic, to use both his social dialect and establishment English, is ignoring current sociological data which depict the negative stereotypes possessed by speakers of such dialects (Williams, 1970).

We see the need for a new professional label, the pediatric language specialist. This specialist is one who is trained in pediatric language development, who can distinguish between linguistic behaviors that are deviant and those that are different, who can teach standard English as a second language, and who can teach developmental language skills or treat defective speech and language patterns using innovative techniques designed to meet the unique needs of different populations.

We believe that these teaching and treating skills distinguish the pediatric language specialist from the more conventional role of the speech-language clinician. Further, a professional who is equipped with these skills would be able to cater more appropriately to the linguistic needs of culturally different and poor children who attend early childhood education programs.

We suggest that the speech-language clinician, in his or her expanded role as a pediatric language specialist, possesses adequate skills to perform a full-time dual function in preschool programs: first, as a speech and language teacher who teaches developmental language skills, and second, as a clinican who treats defective linguistic patterns.

The skills that we would expect the clinician to possess in order to meet the demands of this newly defined role are shown in Fig. 5-1. In addition to meeting the current requirements for certification by the ASHA, the pediatric language specialist will be expected to possess the skills needed to diagnose, teach, and treat developmental speech and language skills to normal preschool children. Notice that implicit in this statement is the assumption that the clinician will be trained to teach dialect speakers establishment or standard English as a second language. To obtain the courses and practica necessary to fulfill these requirements would obviously necessitate a longer period of academic training than is currently required. It is for this reason that specialty certification must be mandated by the ASHA if such training is to be pragmatically possible.

The clinician is also expected to extend the job role beyond the confines of preschool programs by working in conjunction with other professionals in elementary and secondary schools to heighten consciousness as well as to develop appropriate programs and instructional techniques for culturally different and poor children who speak a sociocultural dialect.

When working with very young children, the clinician should be sensitive to the role that parents, teachers, and paraprofessionals play in promoting effective carryover. To realize maximum success in executing these responsibilities, the language specialist should be thoroughly familiar with and utilize properly the Rosenthal effect. Further, the specialist should employ and advocate the use of culture-fair practices in test construction, administration, and interpretation.

The aforementioned tasks are some of the general services which we suggest the pediatric language specialist can and should provide to the children, their parents, and their teachers. More specific suggestions on how to implement various aspects of the new job role are presented at various points throughout this chapter.

III. LANGUAGE DIFFERENCES VERSUS LANGUAGE DEFICITS

The investigation of social dialects in American society has received major impetus in the past decade. The works of Baratz (1969), Dillard (1972), Labov (1966, 1969), Stewart (1967, 1968), Wolfram (1969, 1974) and others have detailed the linguistic regularities not only of Black English but also of the mountain speech of Appalachia. The major conception emerging from this research is that these varieties of English are complete linguistic systems in their own right, with specific rules of grammar, phonology, and lexicon, differing basically in the fact that they are stigmatized or less prestigious forms of standard English (Wolfram and Fasold, 1974).

The following is a brief review of some theoretical explanations of language differences. The review is not intended to be comprehensive, but rather to refresh the reader's knowledge of this information and to present a theoretical framework which forms the basis of this chapter.

There are essentially two diametrically opposed viewpoints relative to the linguistic competence and performance of the culturally different and poor child. One position upholds a deficiency or deficit hypothesis, whereas the other supports a difference hypothesis.

Proponents of the language deficit position, and hence advocates of compensatory education (Bereiter & Engelmann, 1966; Deutsch, 1967; and others) contend that children from so-called deprived backgrounds exhibit thought processes and oral communication skills that are generally inferior to those of middle-class children. Williams (1969) reported that inherent in such literature is the frequent reference made to restrictions and shortcomings in the language development of the poor child. He further stated that a common fallacy in the literature which attempts to support the language deficit theory is that there is a failure to acknowledge that the child is from a different linguistic background, and that the negative attitudes fostered by the teacher toward the child and toward his language result directly in reading difficulty and subsequent failure in school. Williams also emphasized that the language deficit-difference issue is perplexing, in that of the three major professions concerned with describing the language and cognitive abilities of the children (education, psychology, and linguistics) each is assessing the same behavior (the child's oral language production and comprehension) but with varying underlying assumptions; thereby, each sees something different. Some educators purport that the children are essentially verbally destitute; that the children cannot talk, and when they do, their speech is deviant and contaminated with errors. A limited number of psychologists support this position and add that the oral speech of the children is detrimental to cognitive growth. Most linguists and some speech-language clinicians (the current authors included) admonish that these children exhibit linguistic behavior that is different and not deviant; that they speak a well-ordered, highly developed language system which is, in many aspects, different from standard English.

Language differences have been noted in both linguistic and paralinguistic communication patterns as shown in Fig. 5-2. As linguistic differences may occur at the phonological, lexical, or grammatical level, so may paralinguistic variations be reflected in prosodic speech patterns or in aspects of body language. It behooves the speech-language clinician, and particularly the pediatric language specialist, to become knowledgeable about cultural dialects, to recognize the legitimacy of their existence, and to respect the right of the dialect speaker to maintain competence in his or her native dialect. In addition, if possible, the clinician should become conversant in the dialect in order to provide more effective teaching programs and treatment strategies for the children.

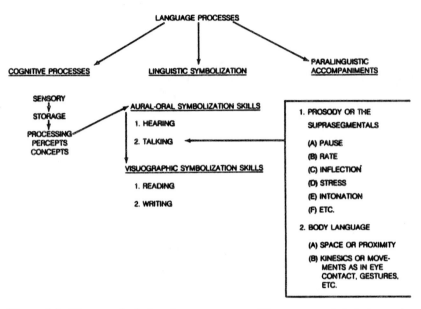

Figure 5-2. Diagram depicting the components of language and their interrelationships.

IV. PRESCHOOL PROGRAMS: HEAD-START AND DAY-CARE-NURSERY SCHOOLS

Currently existing preschool programs such as nursery, day-care, and head-start programs represent training settings in which the services of a pediatric language specialist may be in high demand. The children who attend these programs generally are classified as the economically poor and are often from a cultural background other than middle-class white American. They speak a sociocultural dialect, and they range in age from about 6 months to 5 or 6 years. The majority of the children are in the age range from 3 to 5 years.

The preschool programs may be headed by a director who is usually an early childhood educator; the curriculum is usually designed to prepare the children to meet the minimum entry requirements for first grade.

A number of these requirements focus on the child's ability to speak and understand standard or establishment English as spoken by classroom teachers. Children who enter first grade are expected to be capable of speaking with standard English linguistic patterns and to use and understand the prosodic and kinesic patterns of the standard dialect (see Fig. 5-3).

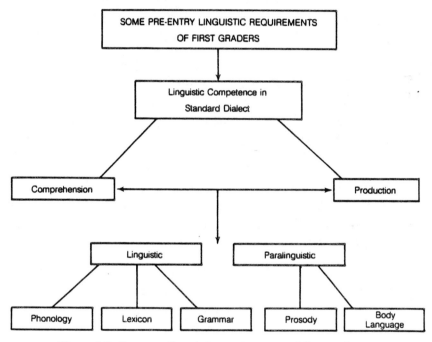

Figure 5-3. Pre-entry linguistic requirements of first graders.

The point is that whereas culturally different and poor children have a language that is sufficient to handle the needs in the home, neighborhood, and peer situations, it is different from the spoken language of the school. Consequently, the child must decode the spoken language of the teacher and make his own language match that of the teacher.

The training programs of many day-care centers employ instructional strategies to meet the socioemotional needs of preschool children while minimizing the amount of formalized teaching to which they are exposed. Essentially, few specific measures are taken to teach the children developmental language skills in these preschool programs.

The fact remains that most of the early education programs continue to embrace misconceptions about the linguistic capabilities of culturally different children. More recently, however, some researchers have begun to promote a growing acceptance of various social dialects as acceptable modes for communicating and learning, and efforts are being made to alter the goals of some school language programs. Instead of attempting to replace child's dialect with standard English, the aim is to design language teaching and treating strategies that will facilitate the development of language skills in both the child's cultural dialect and in standard English.

The ultimate goal of such programs is to increase language skills in general and thereby to enhance the child's ability to code-switch from the cultural dialect to standard English as the situation demands. But who is to teach these skills to children is a question that remains unanswered. Considering that the majority of the children who attend the programs are culturally different and/or economically poor, and usually speak a cultural dialect or language other than standard English, it would seem appropriate to work directly with their aural-oral linguistic skills. The espoused goal would be to provide them with competence in both standard English and the community dialect.

Assuredly, this is one dimension of the role that we envision as being fulfilled by the pediatric language specialist; this worker could *teach* language skills to culturally different and poor children and, concomitantly, *treat* any defective speech and language patterns they might manifest.

We believe that if linguistically different patterns are identified while the children are still very young and standard English is taught as a second language, it may be possible to avert the occurrence of subtle communication problems that may interfere with future educational achievement. The preschool programs that are a part of our discussion provide the ideal setting in which to initiate developmental language intervention programs. Currently, however, these programs are founded on the concepts of compensatory education which involve utilizing a unidialectal-unicultural instructional strategy.

V. COMPENSATORY EDUCATION AND BIDIALECTAL-BICULTURAL TEACHING

A. Compensatory Education

The American school system, predominantly a middle-class institution which teaches middle-class values and ideals from the perspective of middle-class educators, has met with only limited success in educating economically disadvantaged children. Current education programs are based on the assumption that the poor or culturally different child is actually culturally deprived. The goal is to alter the plight of the child by "enriching" his environment or administering a "dose of culture" (Williams, 1969). For the most part, compensatory education is an educational failure for the child. It fosters detrimental psychological and educational effects by attempting to prepare the nonmainstream child for mainstream society, and concomitantly, alienating him from the culture and language of his home and peer community.

In the field of education, the primary determinant of whether or not to continue any program should be its previous record of success. One of the most valid measures of the success of an educational intervention program or method of treatment is whether or not the learner has mastered adequately the skills or educational content to which he or she has been exposed.

At their inception, compensatory programs such as Head-Start were implemented as part of the campaign to enhance the learning abilities and academic performances of poor children. The programs were based upon the so-called malnutrition model, which contends that such children must be force-fed those cognitive nutrients equivalent to the cognitive skills utilized by their middle-class peers. Hence, programs such as Head-Start and early environmental intervention programs including some day-care and nursery school programs were initiated.

An analysis of the educational effectiveness of these programs revealed that they have achieved only minimal success (Hunt, 1969; Jones, 1967; Labov, 1972). Since 1965, the federal government has spent approximately 26 billion dollars under Title I, to "cure" educational disadvantage. Although there have been some successes, most studies conclude such gains as are made are very modest. For example, a Department of Health, Education, and Welfare review of Title

I programs, placed in the Congressional Record in 1977, reviews 10 years of these programs and describes them with labels such as "encouraging"; but no mention is made in this report of significant changes that could be generalized to poor children enrolled in a compensatory program. Labov (1972) pointed out that the fallacy of the compensatory program rests in the fact that educational failures of the child are traced to his personal deficiencies. For instance, Head-Start programs aim to repair the child rather than the school. A program founded on this type of logic inevitably will meet with failure.

B. Bidialectalism

The choices available to educators who teach children with sociocultural dialects are somewhat limited. These include: (1) using only standard English in the classroom; (2) teaching only in the dialect; or (3) utilizing a bidialectal-bicultural approach, or as the case might be, utilizing a multidialectal-multicultural approach.

We are of the opinion that the theoretical framework of bidialectalism provides the best alternative for devising teaching strategies for culturally different children. Briefly, our belief is founded on the following observations. The technique utilized by advocates of compensatory education has generally met with apparently limited success. Programs designed only around the second concept, instruction through dialect, are handicapping to children by failing to expose them to the prestigious "standard" dialect, which is the predominant medium of higher education, business, and government.

In the bidialectal approach, there is a horizontal relationship between the dialect and standard English. This is established by equating dialect and standard English on a functional level, not only teaching children to compare and contrast their own dialect and standard English, but also instructing clinicians and teachers in the crucial concept of "difference." In this approach, the child's cultural-dialectal background is respected and his linguistic horizon is broadened to include an additional language variety.

Implicit in the concept of bidialectalism is the acknowledgment that abstract grammatical knowledge is of no practical value in the actual use of language. The person who is to be educated through the medium of a language or dialect must have more than the ability to phrase sentences or to write rules to generate them as done by modern linguists; he must internalize the rules of that language or dialect so that he uses them automatically. A person who is linguistically competent is one who is capable of using a language appropriately in a variety of social contexts. Communicative competence is exhibited when a person is able to adjust his linguistic code and speech style to conform to the social demands of the situation. Educational endeavors that embrace the concept of teaching standard English by focusing on its form are likely to impede the culturally different child's linguistic competence in standard English and hence to restrict his level of communicative competence.

Labov (1972) and Wolfram (1970) proposed two broad ideas regarding the institutionalization of bidialectalism. Labov mentioned the advantages in first teaching the general items of the different dialects. He recommended that the more general rules should be introduced first in a teaching program. Reportedly, some forms of nonstandard English present special cases in which only one or two words of the language are affected, while there are numerous occurrences of general rules which operate in the nonstandard dialect in consistent ways and can affect the form of every sentence. Additionally, Wolfram (1970) noted the importance of teaching the socially stigmatized variants first in any bidialectal program. We believe that it is certainly easier to determine those features which are generally considered to be nonstandard and socially stigmatizing than to describe the complete nonstandard linguistic system. This philosophy presents a more functional and practical framework from which the teacher-clinician may develop an effective bidialectal program.

Johnson (1971) described five steps that constitute the contrastive analysis approach for bidialectal-bicultural instruction: a child must (1) recognize that there is difference between his language and the language he is learning, (2) hear the target language sound or grammatical pattern, (3) discriminate between his language and the target language at the conflict points, (4) reproduce the target language feature, and (5) practice the target language feature in oral drills. The labels SCHOOL talk and EVERYDAY talk may be used to differentiate between standard English and the child's dialect.

Let us examine how ths relates to the speech-language clinician who is employed in a preschool setting. At this level, special situations may be created to facilitate the discrimination between everyday and school talk. For example, hand puppets may be used early in the program (i.e., an everyday puppet and a school puppet). Later, the clinician may introduce pictures which symbolize a school or everyday environment and require the children to identify various speech patterns as appropriate for each. A more advanced level could involve role-playing; essentially, the child could assume the role of mother, father, teacher, or businessman. A variety of contexts may be used to promote the children's interest and to make the material entertaining so as to retain their attention for longer periods of time.

C. *Biculturalism*

The cultural component of a bidialectal approach for teaching communication skills to the culturally different and poor child involves providing the speakers of varied cultural and linguistic backgrounds with an opportunity to come together as individuals and learn whatever is required in order to function successfully in a multicultural world (Sancho, 1978). In the few settings where a bi-dialectal linguistic teaching and treating approach is utilized, heavy emphasis has been placed on communicative competence (i.e., de-veloping effective diglossic behavior), while the refinement of bi-cultural or multicultural teaching seemingly has been neglected. Sancho (1974) summarized the importance of concomitant bicultural-bidialectal education for culturally different children when he stated: "It is a fact that language cannot be separated from culture; but neither can culture be separated from education, for it is through his cultural background that a student perceives himself, his peers, his school, his teachers, and what education has to offer him"(p. 2).

Central to the concept of bicultural education is the understanding by the teacher that, independent of his background, each child has a plethora of experiences that are meaningful to him and have, to a large degree, shaped him. The teacher-clinician must allow time in the assessment, treatment, and/or instruction plan for every child's viewpoint in order to implement and execute an appropriate and meaningful experience for the child.

The significance of utilizing bicultural or multicultural techniques in our professional encounters with culturally different and poor children can be seen when we adapt instructional methodology that is compatible with the ways in which students are accustomed to learning. This means that as teacher-clinicians we must realize that cognitive or linguistic styles are culturally dependent and not universal. We should accept, understand, appreciate, and respect the fact that individuals of different cultures function as viable and valuable models of legitimate but alternative lifestyles and viewpoints.

A tenable methodology that we feel the teacher-clinician could employ in bicultural or multicultural instruction was discussed by Sancho (1974). He classified cultural elements into two categories; *tangible* and *intangible*. Tangible elements were defined as concrete aspects of a person's culture: those elements which could be taught systematically, such as language, songs, dances, foods, and holidays. Included in the category of intangible elements were items such as values, beliefs, and attitudes held by members of a given cultural group. Apparently these intangibles cannot be taught directly but must be manifested primarily through interpersonal contacts between or among persons of diverse cultural and linguistic backgrounds. Perhaps it is the sharing and exchange of intangible items that hold the key for a viable bicultural or multicultural program at the preschool as well as the more advanced educational levels (i.e., elementary and junior high school programs etc.). Although we do not learn about the values and beliefs of other cultural groups solely through interpersonal contact with them, such close interpersonal encounters serve to enhance our understanding and acceptance of diverse and often opposing viewpoints. The physical setting and composition of the bidialectal-bicultural preschool program (i.e., the Head-Start, day care, or nursery program) provides the unique opportunity for culturally different and poor children as well as for teacher-clinicians of diverse cultural and linguistic backgrounds to experience the close personal interactions that we believe are vital to understanding the intangible aspects of one's culture.

VI. TESTING

Another element of the bidialect-bicultural approach focuses on the assessment and diagnostic procedures that are employed with culturally different and poor children. It is essential that sound testing and test reporting practices be adhered to in this approach.

A vital part of the job description of the pediatric language specialist is to promote culture-fair test assessment and interpretation. In this respect, the clinician can help to guard against possible cultural bias that may be inherent in the construction, administration, and interpretation of test results for poor children. The foundation of the bidialectal language development program is dependent on a reliable and valid interpretation of test results. There are numerous possible sources of cultural bias associated with any standardized test that might invalidate or weaken test results. Some of these are mentioned in the following discussion.

1. A standardized test is most appropriate as an assessment tool for test takers who are most similar to the population on which the test was standardized. The validity of the standardized norm is -weakened when the test is used to assess the performance of culturally different and poor test takers for whom no normative data are provided for comparison. There is no justification for assuming that test takers from different cultural and economic backgrounds perform in the same manner on a particular test. For instance, The Peabody Picture Vocabulary Test (Dunn, 1965), a frequently used assessment device in our profession, was standardized on white, middle-class subjects from Nashville, Tennessee. When the test's standardized norms are used to evaluate scores generated by culturally different and poor children, the tester is being patently unfair. Such a comparison cannot be valid since the culturally different child possesses a receptive vocabulary and linguistic system that is a unique product of his culture, and it is not the same receptive vocabulary and linguistic system of the white middle-class child.

2. Biases may be inherent in the content of some standardized tests. Whenever this occurs, it weakens the validity of the test results since some of the test questions may be dependent upon certain prior experiences which are more familiar to normative groups, usually white, middle-class test takers. Therefore, as Hardy (1976) tells us, incorrect answers do not necessarily indicate incompetence: they may reflect the test taker's unfamiliarity with the content of the test material.

3. Standardized tests may contain biases against the culturally different and poor child created by the situation surrounding test taking. Wolfram and Christian (1976) refer to the test taking procedure as a "social occasion." No matter how well standardized the procedure, these authors contend that the situation surrounding test

taking has cultural contexts.

a. One way in which a testing situation presents cultural variables is that it involves an interaction between a test administrator and a test taker. Severson and Guest (1970) concluded, after a review of research pertaining to examiner difference (including race) and kinds of reinforcement or feedback, that conflicting evidence exists regarding the effects of these variables on culturally different test takers. Their major results were that: "Although it is difficult to make definitive or sweeping statements, the possibility that a number of test-related factors affect test performance of disadvantaged children looms large. Such factors may impair the predictive validity of tests, and the possibility of their influence should be recognized when interpreting test results" (p. 323). Differences in linguistic patterns may affect communication between the culturally different child and the examiner that are subtle, minimal, and not obvious, but significant enough to cause some difficulty in understanding the test directions.

b. Wolfram and Christian (1976) reported that a second factor which relates to the °social occasion" of testing is that it "involves a particular division of labor that distinguishes the testing situation from any other aspect of behavior" (p. 137). In this test situation, the culturally different child may not have the "mind set" for the task at hand that the white, middle-class child is assumed to have.

c. A third variable affecting the culturally different child in the testing situation is the amount of socialization that has taken place prior to the test. The motivational dynamics that affect test behavior are often a function of the pretest relationship between the tester and the child. When that relationship is characterized by an informal and "healthy" interaction, the child is more likely to be motivated to perform at his best.

Test Reporting

For clinical purposes, the clinician should interpret a culturally biased test by (a) reporting the test results with reference to the population on which the test was standardized, and (b) reporting the test results with reference to the child's cultural peer group. This necessitates detailing those dialect-specific forms that the child used in his test response which are acceptable forms in his dialect speech community.

Similarly, for educational purposes, the clinician should again interpret the results in terms of the culturally different child's middle-class peers on which the test was standardized — since the child must function in an educational system which is based on similar middle-class principles — however, emphasizing the cultural biases inherent in this approach. In addition the clinician should describe the child's performance in comparison to his or her peers in the dialect speech community.

Finally, it would be helpful if the clinician could ascertain some measure of the child's diglossic skills in order to make some reasonable projections regarding his or her ability to understand and use the standard dialect spoken in the schools.

VII. PROGRAMMING FOR DEVELOPMENTAL LANGUAGE

A crucial concept in this chapter is that the speech and language patterns of many culturally different and poor children are sufficiently different from standard English to make their comprehension often difficult for standard English speakers. Frequently, the nonstandard speaker's use of standard English patterns with his peer group may result in communication breakdowns, conflict with peers, and/or ridicule by his peers. As a consequence, the child is often poorly motivated to utilize standard English. We suggest that one way to resolve this problem is to train the child to be diglossic (i.e., to use standard English in the school and in his social interactions with standard English speakers, and to use nonstandard dialect in his social environment with peers and other nonstandard dialect speakers).

Ideally, we suggest introducing the child to standard English during the preschool years because these years are critical to grammatical development, particularly during the years from approximately 2½ to 5 years of age (Meers, 1976). Moreover, it is generally established that the child is more adept at learning a second language during the preschool years than in later years. It follows that the preschool years would be an appropriate time to explore the possibility of teaching a second language. In this manner, the child's linguistic and paralinguistic behavior can be expanded to include both the knowledge of when to code-switch and the necessary linguistic and paralinguistic skills to be communicatively diglossic. This we contend, is a more practical solution than attempting to eradicate the child's native dialect by instructing him or her only in standard English dialect and rejecting and ridiculing the child's cultural dialect (which is usually the case in the desegregated classroom that enrolls children from a variety of sociolinguistic and socioeconomic backgrounds). In addition, institutionalization of the Rosenthal effect in such programs may serve to enhance the automatic utilization of "school language" or standard English dialect by the time the child enters elementary school. Of course, presently, this represents some conjecture on the part of the authors, but our position is supported by research being conducted by the senior author.* As was mentioned previously, in the Rosenthal effect, people alter their behavior in the manner they perceive the investigator wants them to change. Research on dialectally different speech patterns has revealed that nonstandard cultural dialects may differ from standard English on a variety of linguistic levels including the phonological, lexical, and syntactical levels. Furthermore, differences may exist between the paralinguistic features that characterize the two dialects (i.e., differences in prosody and body language). If we acknowledge that these communicative patterns simply may represent "differences" and not "deficiencies" (while some dialectal patterns may be both different and deficient) and that the current medium of instruction in the school system is the standard English dialect, then it behooves speech-language clinicians to reexamine the assessment, treating, and teaching strategies that they employed in their interactions with dialect speakers. Specifically, they need to evaluate critically the current practice to label and treat as "deficient" those utterances which differ from our standard English equivalent. We believe that as speech-language clinicians, and preferably as "communicologists," we should become more integrally involved in planning and implementing bidialectal-bicultural programs to teach these children an alternate form of communication (i.e., standard English, beginning at the preschool level). We should prepare ourselves to assume the role of communicologists; that is, one who is involved totally with the child's communication development, including planning and implementing appropriate and effective assessment, teaching, and

---

*The reader is referred to our 2-year research program with Head-Start children: for copies of this research write to the senior author.

treating strategies that will, in effect, enhance diglossic development in dialect speakers.

Another component of effective programming that should be developed involves incorporating facilitative programs with teachers, paraprofessionals, and parents. We realize that in different, but important, ways each of these support groups can be instrumental in facilitating the communicative needs of all children who receive the services of the pediatric language specialist. To achieve this goal, we encourage the teacher-clinician to design and implement programs with families and teachers to educate them about language differences.

Previous experience with these groups has shown that parent groups of culturally different and poor children often present the most resistive attitudes toward accepting the concept of "difference." This reaction is not surprising, since it is the parents who have been stigmatized and penalized socially and economically for years because they speak a sociocultural dialect. These parents do not want their children to be subject to the same attack. The fact is that they want their children to be able to speak the establishment dialect (i.e., "good" English), and they depend on the schools to accomplish this goal.

It is not our intention to suggest that teachers and paraprofessional aides readily accept the propriety of a cultural dialect. Rather, they too are reluctant to acknowledge the legitimacy of cultural dialects. This attitude is not surprising either; for years we have all been taught that there is only one "correct" way to talk and that is to use standard English as spoken by the classroom teacher. Fortunately, our experience with parents, teachers, and paraprofessionals over the past few years has shown that their attitudes are amenable to change. Obviously, this implies the need to develop educational programs for these groups. The following suggestions may be helpful:

A. Suggestions for Working with Parents

1. Ascertain from parents, via a carefully constructed questionnaire, exactly how they feel about the way they talk and about their children's speech patterns.
2. Instruct parents about the concept of "difference."
3. Instruct parents regarding the nature of bidialectalism and

biculturalism. Ascertain their understanding and acceptance of the concepts.

4. Design specific exercises that parents can engage in either individually or collectively. These exercises should involve examples of standard dialect contrasted with examples of the cultural dialect as spoken by the parents (from tape recordings). Allow parents a chance to hear both versions and to become comfortable with the concept that both versions are correct and appropriate ways of talking in the respective dialects.

5. Provide parents with concrete ideas that may be implemented in the home to promote carryover from their child's bidialectal program in the school.

6. Let parents know that you realize the important role that they play (as the person who spends the most time with the child) in the total development of the child. Emphasize the importance of their participation in the carryover phase of the bidialectal program.

7. Provide parents with periodic feedback updating them on the performance of their child in the program. In addition, let them know directly how effective you feel they have been in helping to promote the child's success. (A short tape recording of some of the children as they talk in the classroom and on the playground may elicit positive reactions from parents.)

8. Provide parents with periodic in-service training. Start by including an interaction session during the regularly scheduled, monthly parent-teacher meetings. These sessions need not last more than 15 or 20 minutes. Plan the sessions so that parents are provided educational instruction on bidialectalism as well as on practical application of concepts. Be sure to encourage verbal exchange among parents regarding their attitudes toward the concepts and the experiences they and their children have shared since the initiation of the program in the schools.

B. Suggestons for Working with Teachers

Help the teacher to design a developmental language program that the child enjoys and looks forward to each day:

1. Give the child reasons to be proud of his dialect by educating him regarding its history and origin.
2. Provide the child with evidence of acceptance and respect for his language difference by positively reinforcing him when he uses the dialect in the appropriate situation.
3. Allow the child opportunities to "see" how the dialect is equivalent to standard English by providing him with illustrative contrasts between the two dialects and explaining when it is appropriate to use the different versions of communication.
4. Avoid using terms such as "correct," "incorrect," "right," or "wrong" when referring to the child's dialect or standard English. Rather, choose terms such as "school" talk and "everyday" talk (or "street" talk, etc.). The goal is to eliminate any implication that standard English is the correct way to talk and that the dialectal version is the incorrect way to talk.
5. Reward the child for his use of standard English (or the dialect as the case may be) in situations other than the formal language teaching and treating sessions. For example, "I am really proud of the way you are using school talk while we are working your math problems today"; or "You have really learned to switch from school talk to everyday talk quite well!"

VIII. PARALINGUISTICS

Another important phase of the language development program that is usually neglected by the speech-language clinician involves planning and implementing a sound paralinguistic component. We should prepare ourselves to teach and treat features of paralinguistic behavior concomitant with our teaching and treating of linguistic behaviors. This need becomes more evident if we examine briefly some of the research that has evolved in this area.

Recently, researchers in the area of human behavior have begun to investigate and specify the significance of paralinguistic features in the role of effective communication and/or normal linguistic development (Mehrabian, 1969; Wood, 1976). Paralinguistic features include body language, prosodic features, and other nonlinguistic features such as voice quality and vocal reflexes. Wood (1976) indicated that young children communicate in a very physical manner;

that is, they frequently point, nod, wave, etc. when they talk. As children develop verbal skills, the bodily channel of communication becomes more entwined in the total communication process. Wood (1976) described body language as including "all reflexive and non-reflexive movements and positions of the body that communicate emotional, attitudinal and informational messages" (p. 204). Just as children learn the phonology, grammar, and lexicon of their language, they must also learn the patterns of bodily movements that communicate messages to others.

Prosodic features, on the other hand, are perhaps the earliest dimension of language to be used and understood by young children. Prosody is the critical marking that makes one's speech uniquely his own. The prosody of speech is flexible, varying with our moods, thoughts, and feelings. The components of prosody (pitch, loudness, pause, intonation, rhythm, etc.) are altered to produce meaningful signals in our messages. The intricate interaction among these elements results in an exceedingly complex vocal system (Mehrabian, 1969; Wood, 1976).

Generally, speech-language specialists and others have considered that the major channel of communication is by the linguistic transmission of information. On the contrary, nonlinguistic communication systems, including body language and prosodic features, are of fundamental importance in the interpretation of a message and its impact upon the auditor. Both linguistic and paralinguistic components operate in a synchronized, coordinated fashion in human communication, and the nonverbal components of a message may either confirm or contradict the verbal message (Mehrabian, 1969; Wood, 1976).

Mehrabian (1969) proposed a formula to project the interaction among the linguistic symbols, body language, and prosody in effective communication. He proposed that the verbal portion of the message contributes about 7% of the total impact of the message, the prosodic or suprasegmental portion about 38%, and facial expression, a facet of body language, about 55%. This shows that, contrary to traditional beliefs regarding the important role of the verbal portion of a message, the prosodic and facial cues are the most essential in influencing an auditor's attitude toward a speaker in face-to-face situations.

Until quite recently, only minimal importance has been attached to the systematic investigation and quantification of the paralinguistic aspects of language patterns of the culturally different and poor (for example, see Westbrook, 1975). By tradition, sociolinguists and clinicians alike have concentrated primarily on describing the segmental features of social dialects, de-emphasizing study of suprasegmental feature differences. However, since language communication involves the use of both linguistic and paralinguistic components, it follows logically that there is a need for more systematic and detailed documentation of those paralinguistic features that distinguish the dialects.

A commonly reported result in the existing research is that differences between the body langauge and prosodic features of nonstandard English speakers and standard English speakers are significant enough to create communication breakdowns (Adler, 1979; Tarone, 1973; Westbrook, 1975; Winkler, 1975). Thus, it is incumbent upon teachers and clinicians to become knowledgeable about culturally dominated patterns of body language and prosody which may be encountered in their interactions with culturally different and poor children.

Some research has revealed that posture and body movement, facial displays, and various suprasegmental features (such as speech rhythm and intonation patterns, and syllabication and stress patterns) may assume different and important roles in communicating among different cultures. For example, Flen (cited in Adler, 1979) reported that postural stance is well recognized as an important means of projecting self-image among Black males, whereas a guarded and slow-moving movement pattern is more prominent among Appalachians.

From a bidialectal standpoint, the culturally different and poor child should be provided with the facility to switch not only segmental codes but suprasegmental codes as well. Furthermore, the speech-language clinician should develop adequate skills that will enable him or her to make valid judgments about the appropriateness of the suprasegmental features of the dialect speaker.

Of necessity, this entails developing a bicultural orientation in which the teacher-clinician becomes functionally knowledgeable about the role of suprasegmentals in the dialect community language. Recognizing that limited groundwork has been laid in this area, the teacher-clinician can begin by obtaining tape-recorded samples of the dialect speech in a particular geographic region and practice developing the perceptual skills for recognizing the dialect-specific features. In addition, he or she should become cognizant of the suprasegmental features of the standard dialect of that region. This will enable him to become more familiar with the standard dialect's equivalent suprasegmental feature(s) and thereby to form the necessary basis for designing contrastive ear-training strategies.

Accurate record keeping will enable the clinician to specify those suprasegemental features that are important for that dialect speech community. Also of primary importance is the acknowledgment that the language of the culturally different speaker will vary with geographic region. Thus, the features of prosody that characterize one dialect speech community may differ slightly from those of another community.

Another method of acquiring the necessary data and increasing the skills of the clinician is through the sharing of clinical information among peer professionals. In a given geographic region clinicians may collect data over a particular period of time and collate the information, thereby obtaining a more representative sample of the variable being studied (i.e., prosodic feature differences).

Clinicians must therefore equip themselves to evaluate the suprasegmental features of the dialect speaker's speech, just as they have obtained extensive skills in describing and evaluating the segmental features of standard English and, more recently, but without as much consistency, those of Black English and Mountain English. Consequently, more accurate judgments regarding the "difference or deficiency" of the child's suprasegmental features can be made and appropriate teaching or treating strategies can be implemented.

What are the implications of this discussion to the clinicians who will be responsible for treating or teaching language to the poor child? Perhaps the most obvious one is that clinicians must arm themselves with the necessary knowledge and expertise to evaluate the total communicative abilities of all children, not just of the culturally different or poor child. This entails attaining certain levels of proficiency in the understanding of both the linguistic and paralinguistic features of language. It further involves an understanding of the interrelation of *linguistic symbols, body language,* and *prosody.* As mentioned earlier, Mehrabian (1969) devised a formula which he felt depicts how the three communicative components interact to convey a particular message to a receiver. This relationship clearly indicates that in face-to-face interactions, people are more dependent on prosodic and facial cues than on linguistic content in determining another's attitude toward them (i.e., the intended impact of the message). It is critical that speech-language clinicians learn to recognize and understand these paralinguistic features in order to ensure effective communication with their clients. We cannot emphasize this enough.

Finally, any approach that is used to teach prosodic features, i.e., intonation and stress (from a bidialectal standpoint) must reflect the language and experiences (cultural) of the learner (i.e., culturally different and poor child). The foundation of such a program should focus on contrasting and comparing the nonstandard feature with its standard English feature or equivalent. Again, this might involve the use of the terms school talk and everyday talk to illustrate the contrasts more vividly.

Suprasegmental Features: Teaching Ideas

1. Build lessons around such TV programs as "Fat Albert." Have child(ren) watch the program and remember examples of everyday talk that were used. Either have the child supply the school talk equivalent or supply it for them. This program provides numerous examples of suprasegmental differences as well as of segmental differences.
2. Record the speech of various diglossic culturally different speakers depicting their production which includes dialectal stress patterns and intonational patterns and the standard dialect contrast or equivalent stress and intonation patterns.
3. Record the speech of the child(ren) as he (they) speaks formally and informally to be used later in ear-training and contrast exercises.

IX. SELF-CONCEPT AND
THE ROSENTHAL EFFECT

We can assume that the amount and kind of learning that a child experiences greatly influence the way he feels about himself, his peers, and the classroom environment. The child with a positive self-concept has a fairly realistic view of his strengths and weaknesses and generally is accepted by his peers. Usually, the child with a negative self-concept has an unrealistic view of his strengths and weaknesses that is associated with his direct experiences with failure and the ambivalence in the feedback he receives from those around him regarding his strengths and weaknesses.

Children with impaired self-concepts may or may not possess the skills or competence which they are convinced they do not have. A poor self-concept is characterized by persistent self-criticism and low self-esteem. For obvious reasons, problems in self-concept are critical in the education of culturally different and poor children. This group of children is prone to be regarded negatively by teachers and peers simply because of the unwarranted stigmata that tend to be associated with being poor. Sometimes, though not always, the personal hygiene of these children may be less than desirable, or the children may be distinguished by such trivial characteristics as their wearing apparel, or, more importantly, by their dialectal speech patterns. While we are all aware of the biases inherent in stereotyping any group of people based solely upon our limited knowledge of the cultural institutions of these people, the temptation to harbor such biases still exists.

The attitude that teacher-clinicians manifest toward a child will ultimately affect the feeling that that child fosters about himself. The fact is that a child must feel good about himself in order to profit maximally from the educational experience; such a positive self-concept certainly enhances the learning process. The pediatric language specialist is in a key position to influence the social-emotional behavior, the feelings, and the attitudes of the learner. The behavior that the clinician shows toward the child can significantly affect acceptance of that particular child by his peers. Moreover, the teacher's attitude can affect the child's performance in the classroom.

Most of us are familiar with the term "self-fulfilling prophesy." The self-fulfilling prophesy has been used by Rosenthal and Jacobson (1968) to describe the effects of teacher expectancy on pupil performance. The point is made that one reason for the poor academic performance of children using a different dialect is that a poor performance is expected of them. A child's shortcomings may originate not in his different ethnic, cultural, economic, and linguistic background, but in the teacher's response to the child's background.

A study (Rosenthal & Jacobson, 1968) was performed in which the majority of students were children from lower-class families, whose parents were receiving welfare aid, and were of Mexican origin. The participants were pre- and posttested at the beginning and end of the school year with instruments that measured verbal and reasoning abilities. Teachers were informed early in the school term that certain children were "spurters," who actually were selected at random. Results showed that spuriously labeling certain children as potentially gifted resulted in a dramatic incline in their posttest ability scores (i.e., the Rosenthal effect). The difference of 15 IQ points on posttests is almost equivalent to the amount of lag reported for culturally different children. Essentially, encouraging teachers to consider any such children as "special" from a positive perspective resulted in eradicating the deficit usually associated with low socioeconomic status. The most obvious explanation for the rise in the posttest ability scores is that the teachers spent more time with these particular children. However, Rosenthal and Jacobson (1968) purported that the explanations seem to lie in a subtle feature of the interaction of the teachers and pupils. The suggestion was that the tone of voice, facial expression, touch, and posture assumed by the teachers may be the means by which they communicated expectations to pupils. Thus, effective communication may have been influential in changing children's self-concepts, their anticipation of their own behaviors, and their motivation to enhance their cognitive skills. These changes were than reflected in the posttest scores.

The study by Rosenthal and Jacobson illustrates how a person's behavior tends to be dependent, to a considerable degree, upon the person's perception of what others expect of him or her as well as the attitude (subtle or overt) that is conveyed to the person by important authorities. Therefore, knowledge of the Rosenthal effect is especially relevant to pediatric language specialists in their interactions with the culturally different and poor. Whether it is purposely or not, those who are culturally dissimilar from the clinician or the teacher tend to receive less attention; and we tend to foster lower performance expectations of them than of those who share a cultural background similar to the authority figure. Williams (1969) noted that a teacher has certain evaluational reactions to a student's speech, which are stereotyped versions of his attitudes toward the speaker. He implied that the teacher bases much of his instructional behavior toward a pupil upon that stereotyped attitude. Thus a child's speech may serve as an indication of his cultural background, and when the teacher encounters a culturally different child perhaps subconsciously he expects nonstandardness, reticence, and uncertainty from the child. Similarly, the child may have acquired reciprocal stereotyped and negative attitudes toward the teacher. It follows that teacher-pupil interactions are affected by teacher-pupil expectations. If a teacher treats a child as if he were reticent, insecure, and a product of that which is substandard, the child will react in a similar manner. He will harbor the feeling that he, and all that he represents, is inferior because others judge his language behavior as inferior. The culturally different and poor child may experience frustration and educational alienation because he must acquire his education in an unfamiliar and unnatural language.

The pediatric language specialist is one who is trained to be cognizant of the detrimental effects that negative teacher attitudes and expectations may have upon a child's self-concept as well as upon his social and academic performance. The specialist should strive, therefore, to create an atmosphere of acceptance and of mutual respect that will promote a positive self-concept in all children.

In addition, one should realize that in order for the child to be successful in developing a more positive concept about himself, including the legitimacy and appropriateness of his dialect and his diglossic behavior, he must also receive support and approval from his community. For this reason, an effective parent education program may be invaluable. As mentioned previously, parents should be made fully aware of the goals of our developmental language teaching and treating program. Essentially, in order for the program to be a complete success, parents must also revise their thinking with respect to their children's speech behavior.

X. SUMMARY STATEMENT

An alteration is recommended in the job description of the speech-language clinician. Not only should he or she treat communicatively disordered clients, but also teach developmental language skills to preschool children — particularly poor children in day-care or other preschool centers. To accomplish this, specialty certification in the American Speech Language and Hearing Association must become workable.

We envision a new breed of speech-language clinician in the immediate future. The change that we foresee in our current job description is a result of many changes including (1) the increase in the numbers of recently graduated clinicians who are entering the job market and the difficulties to be encountered in finding positions in conventional programs; (2) the impact of recently enacted legislation; for instance, the *Education for all Handicapped Children Act* (Public Law 94-142) which requires changes in teaching and treating methods in order to comply fully with the law; and (3) the expansion in the female work-force (the latest estimate is that approximately half of the married female population is currently employed in out-of-home activities) will inevitably cause the number of day-care facilities to increase. A basic function of such programs should be to enhance the communicative skills of children: acceptable academic acquisition must ultimately rest upon an appropriate language base. It has been our intent in this chapter to provide those concepts relevant to such language programs; in particular, the pluralistic philosophy undergirding any developmental program for poor children.

Our work with the Pediatric Language Institutes (PLI) program, a facet of our Pediatric Language Programs at the University of Tennessee, has documented how important such a program can be to day-care center personnel. If we, as professionals, do not wish to become actively involved in the direction of such centers, it is at least incumbent upon us to offer guidance to day-care center workers. The results of the PLI program can attest to the efficacy of such advisory relationships. Furthermore, to direct such programs, as we do in our Pediatric Language Laboratory program — a day-care center which we maintain on the University of Tennessee campus — is a rewarding experience for the pediatric language specialist.

There is an existing need for such involvement. Speech-language clinicians should cater to this need.

REFERENCES

Adler, S. Dialectal Speech: Professional and Clinical-Implications. *Journal of*

Speech and Hearing Disorders, 1971, 36, 90-100.

Adler, S. Data Gathering: The Reliability and Validity of Test Data from Culturally Different Children. *Journal of Learning Disabilities,* 1973, 6, 30-35.

Adler, S. *Poverty Children and Their Language: Implications for Teaching and Treating.* New York: Grune & Stratton, 1979.

Baratz, J. Teaching Reading in An Urban Negro School System. In J. Baratz and R. Shuy (Eds.), *Teaching Black Children to Read.* Washington, D.C.: Center for Applied Linguistics, 1969. pp. 92-116.

Bereiter, C., & Engelmann, S. *Teaching Disadvantaged Children in the Preschool.* Englewood Cliffs, N.J.: Prentice-Hall, 1966.

Deutsch, C. P. Auditory Discrimination and Learning. In M. Deutsch *et al.* (Eds.), *The Disadvantaged Child.* New York: Basic Books, 1967. pp. 259-277.

Dillard, J. L. *Black English: Its History and Usage in the United States.* New York: Random House, 1972.

Dunn, L. M. *The Peabody Picture Vocabulary Test.* Circle Pines, Minn.: American Guidance Service, 1965.

Hardy, J., Welcher D., Mellits E., & Kagan J. Pitfalls in the Measurement of Intelligence: Are Standardized Intelligence Tests Valid Instruments for Measuring the Intellectual Potential of Urban Children? *Journal of Psychology,* 94, 1976, 43-51.

Hunt, J. M. *The Challenge of Incompetence and Poverty.* Chicago: University of Illinois Press, 1969.

Johnson, K. R. Should Black Children Learn Standard English? In M. Imhoof (Ed.), *Social Educational Insights into Teaching Standard English to Speakers of Other Dialects.* Bloomington, Ind.: Indiana University Press, 1971. pp. 83-101.

Jones, J. P. *Child Development.* Austin, Texas: Head-Start Evaluation and Research Center, 1967.

Labov, W. *The Social Stratification of English in New York City.* Washington, D.C.: Center for Applied Linguistics, 1966.

Labov, W. Some Sources of Reading Problems for Negro Speakers of Nonstandard English. In J. Baratz & R. Shuy (Eds.), *Teaching Black Children to Read.* Washington, D.C.: Center for Applied Linguistics, 1969. pp. 29-67.

Labov, W. *Language in the Inner City: Studies in the Black English Vernacular.* Philadelphia: University of Pennsylvania Press, 1972.

Meers, H. J. *Helping Our Children Talk.* London: Longmans, 1976.

Mehrabian, A. Communication Without Words. In *Readings in Psychology Today.* Del Mar, Cal.: CMR Books, 1969, pp. 276-279.

Rosenthal, R., & Jacobson, L. F. Teacher Expectations for the Disadvantaged. *Scientific American,* 1968, 218, 19-23.

Severson, R., & Guest, K. Toward the Standardized Assessment of the Language of Disadvantaged Children. In F. Williams (Ed.). *Language and Poverty.* Chicago: Markham, 1970. pp. 309-355.

Sancho, A. R. Culture in the Bilingual-bicultural Curriculum. *ERIC Document 096814,* March, 1974. pp. 1-12.

Stewart, W. A. Continuity and Change in American Negro Dialects. *Florida Foreign Language Reporter,* 1968, 6, 3-4, 14-16, 18.

Stewart, W. A. Sociolinguistic Factors in the History of American Negro Dialects. The *Florida Foreign Language Reporter,* 1967, 5, 11, 22, 24, 26.

Tarone, E. Aspects of Intonation in Black English. *ERIC Document 076983,* September, 1973. pp. 2-12.

Westbrook, C. R. Suprasegmental Aspects of Reading Interference. *ERIC Document 117691,* April, 1975, pp. 2-10.

Williams, E. *On the Contribution of the Linguist to Institutional Racism.* Paper presented at the convention of the Linguistic Society of America, San Franciso, 1969.

Williams, F., Language, Attitude, and Social Change. In F Williams (Ed.), *Language and Poverty.* Chicago: Markham Publishing Company, 1970. pp. 380-399.

Winkler, J. H. A Comparison of the Intonation Patterns of Black English and Standard English. *ERIC Document 096813,* February, 1976, pp. 2-7.

Wolfram, W. A. *Sociolinguistic Description of Detroit Negro Speech.* Washington, D.C.: Center for Applied Linguistics, 1969.

Wolfram, W. Sociolinguistic Implications for Educational Sequencing. In R. Fasold & R. Shuy (Eds.), *Teaching Standard English in the Inner City.* Washington, D.C.: Center for Applied Linguistics, 1970, pp. 105-119.

Wolfram, W. On the Relationship of Sociolinguistics and Speech Pathology. *ERIC Document 135242,* December, 1976, pp. 2-23.

Wolfram, W. & Christian, D., *Appalachian Speech.* Washington, D.C.: Center for Applied Linguistics, 1976.

Wolfram, W. & Fasold, R. *The Study of Social Dialects in American English.* Englewood Cliffs, N.J.: Prentice-Hall, 1974.

Wood, B. S. *Children and Communication: Verbal and Non-verbal Language Development.* Englewood Cliffs, N.J.: Prentice-Hall, 1976.

Chapter VI

ISSUES IN LAYPERSON BIAS TOWARD THE CULTURAL DIFFERENCE VIEW

SANDRA L. TERRELL

"She wouldn't have a very good job 'cause they would think she wasn't very smart" *(A 12-year old child commenting on the kind of job he thought a dialect-speaker might have).*

EACH profession probably has some obvious, recurring problems with which its practitioners must individually deal in the best way they can since the problems have never been addressed in a systematic way. As an example of such a circumstance within the profession of communication disorders, the issue of dialectal variation among adult minorities has not been researched despite the high prevalence of stroke-related language disorders among blacks (Holland, 1983). Yet another topic relevant to speech and language experts that has been largely neglected is the issue of linguistic and cultural bias among laypersons. Layperson bias concerns the problems that language specialists are confronted with when members of the general public have failed to accept the legitimacy of the normal linguistic variations of English (i.e., social

The author wishes to gratefully acknowledge the speech-language pathologists who graciously and courageously shared their personal experiences and insights.

119

dialects). An additional aspect of layperson bias may include the immediate assumption by various members of the public that the minority professional is probably less capable than the non-minority professional. Still another type of layperson bias is that speech and language professionals of any ethnicity who choose to provide services primarily to low income and various minority groups may be perceived to be less fortunate than professionals who provide clinical services to affluent individuals.

Laypersons include parents, relatives, neighborhood children, employment managers, and everyone else outside the realm of speech and language experts who are able to consciously or unconsciously discriminate between standard and non-standard varieties of English and react differentially toward the speech patterns and other characteristics of various ethnic and social groups.

It is emphasized that there is no research available to substantiate the prevalence of layperson bias, and only one study is available that suggests that layperson bias currently exists (Terrell and Terrell, 1983). However, based on the experiences of speech-language pathologists, other language specialists, and social dialect speakers that have been shared with me after hours at professional meetings, over lunch, during coffee breaks at in-services, and at community functions, there is some rudimentary evidence that incidents of layperson bias are common occurrences which could interfere with clinical service efficacy. Based upon this rudimentary evidence and some scant literature, there seems to be at least three types of layperson bias. These include 1) societal bias toward speakers of non-standard varieties of English; 2) bias toward minority speech-language pathologists, audiologists, and other language specialists; and 3) bias toward experts who choose to provide clinical services to low income and various minority populations.

The purpose of this essay is to illustrate the various problems that may arise from layperson bias and how these problems might be best managed. Two female speech-language pathologists separately recounted their experiences with layperson bias and how they resolved the situations. One speech-language pathologist is white and has provided clinical services to a predominately black middle school in a southwestern area for the past five years. She is currently employed in this same position. The other professional is a black speech-language pathologist who provided clinical services to two rural southern elementary schools seven years ago. She has since relocated to another geographic area where she currently supervises speech-language pathology students at a moderately large, multiethnic university. Transcriptions of the accounts of these two professionals will be provided as examples of the types of layperson bias that can occur. Based upon these accounts, some interim management principles and caveats to layperson bias management will be offered. An additional section of the paper will provide background literature relevant to the topic.

BACKGROUND

Few professionals who specialize in speech and language are unaware of the dialectal deficiency-difference battle that has existed over the past two decades. In review, the debate was between two contrasting theories that were postulated to explain the linguistic characteristics between black and white children. On the one hand, some theorists argued that lower socioeconomic and various ethnic groups have a language deficiency. Theorists espousing this deficiency hypothesis held the view that black children tend to use fewer words than middle-class white children and that this performance reflects a cognitive deficiency (Deutsch, 1965; John, 1963; Bereiter and Engelmann, 1966; Osser, Wang, and Zaid, 1969). In contrast, Labov (1966), Shuy (1969), and Baratz (1969) have argued that a legitimate dialectal difference exists among the various ethnic groups. These theorists suggested that variations in linguistic style found among various ethnic groups reflect cultural differences.

The linguistic controversy stimulated many articles on the subject in support of the difference hypothesis. Additional studies have provided evidence that is inconsistent with the deficiency interpretation. Studies in support of the difference interpretation have typically demonstrated that systematic phonologic, morphologic, and discourse patterns exist among various social varieties of American English (Williams and Wolfram, 1977; Houston, 1970; Kochman, 1971; Taylor, 1982; Williams, 1981). Other studies have provided data to refute the deficiency interpretation. In general these studies adjusted procedures to account for cultural factors that are relevant to black children. These studies demonstrate that when cultural factors are accounted for, there are no significant differences between black and white children on various linguistic and cognitive measures (Terrell, 1975; Terrell, Terrell, and Golin, 1977). Due to the efforts of these authors, there is now widespread acceptance among language specialists that the linguistic style common among various cultural groups is a viable communicative system. For example, this viewpoint was recently adopted by the American Speech-Language-Hearing Association as the official policy on social dialects for its 36,000 members (*Asha*, September, 1983).

The victory of the difference theorists, while noteworthy, has also resulted in new problems which require attention. One of these problems concerns exactly how dialect speakers should be managed within educational and clinical settings. Acceptance of the difference view does not automatically make a professional knowledgeable about how to appropriately respond when there is a need to provide services to a dialect speaker. Due to the focus of previous dialect studies, which was to provide credibility to the difference viewpoint, literature regarding techniques for the most effective management of dialect speakers is just becoming more frequent in the literature.

For example, one of the first publications to apply the difference model to the practical management of black children is edited by Baratz and Shuy (1969). This book contains articles by various authors in order to share information on more effective ways educators can use to teach black children how to read. In general, these authors state that initial reading skills must be developed based upon the child's existing dialect.

Additional authors have provided strategies for resolving bias problems in the language and cognitive assessment of black children (Seymour and Miller-Jones, 1981; Butler and Terrell, 1983). As a final example of the increasing literature on management of the dialect speaker, Holland (1983) has provided several common-sense principles for the non-discriminatory assessment of minority adults with language disorders. These articles, taken collectively, suggest that authors are extending beyond the deficiency-difference debate and are sharing information on how non-discriminatory clinical services for members of various minority and ethnic groups can best be accomplished.

Another problem has also emerged from the resolution of the old linguistic controversy. This problem does not concern the bias of language professionals in their services for various minority and ethnic minorities. Rather, this problem concerns the bias of laypersons toward dialect speakers and toward the language professionals who provide clinical services to these speakers. Apparently, the experts who have accepted the legitimacy of social dialects and strive to provide nondiscriminatory patient care delivery have yet to convince the public to also accept this stance.

Language variation has been attributed to several factors. Among these factors include race and ethnicity, social class, education, occupation, and geographical region (Taylor, 1982). There is evidence to suggest that a combination of these factors contributes to language diversity more so than one factor alone (Terrell, 1975).

Additional literature provides evidence that laypersons not only recognize such linguistic diversities, but react differentially toward them. Kutner, Wilkins, and Yarrow (1952) investigated the reactions of 11 restaurant managers toward letters requesting reservations for a social gathering of people, some of whom were black. After more than two weeks without a reply, follow-up phone calls to each restaurant were made reminding each restaurant manager of the letter and requesting reservations. The follow-up phone calls were made by one of two white women. No managers accepted the telephone reservations for the racially mixed group. However, all managers accepted reservations for a control phone call made by the same person who made the first follow-up call. The control call asked for reservations for a group of friends without any reference to the racial composition of the group. Although the race of the caller was not a main factor of the study, the use of the white caller as opposed to a black person indicates that the researchers saw race of caller as a confounding variable that was necessary to control. Less valid results may have been obtained if the restaurant managers had perceived the caller as black.

In a more recent study, Terrell and Terrell (1983) investigated the reactions of personnel managers to standard English and Black English speakers. Two groups of black females applied for secretarial positions advertized in newspapers of a large southwestern city. One group spoke primarily Black English and the other group spoke standard English. It was found that Black English speakers were offered fewer jobs than the standard English speakers were, and when these non-standard English speakers were offered positions, it was at a significantly lower salary than that offered to standard English speakers. This research thus provides evidence that misconceptions and biases may continue to exist among laypersons in this current decade.

Other studies indicate that differential reactions toward linguistic diversity exist in children as young as preschool age. Rosenthal (1974) asked preschool children to decide which of two boxes they preferred to take a present from and which of the boxes they wanted to give a present to. The boxes were decorated into identical faces in colors that did not represent or imply any racial group. Via remote-control cassettes hidden behind each box, one box tried to persuade the child using standard English and the other box used Black English. After listening to both boxes, each child was asked a series of questions regarding his/her choice of a box to take a present from and which box the child wished to give a present to. In general, the children preferred to take their presents from the standard English-speaking box. The children perceived that the standard English-speaking box had better presents than the dialect-speaking box. (The presents, which were crayons, were identical for both boxes.) Although the children felt that the black English-speaking box needed a present more, most of the children gave the present (a pad of paper) to the standard English-speaking box. These results suggest that young children are not only aware of dialect differences, but also develop opinions about dialect speakers at an early age.

A recent pilot study offers further evidence that differential reactions toward various social dialects exists among laypersons. Terrell (1981) tape recorded two versions of an explanation on how to keep cool in the summer (see Appendix). The explanation differed only in the dialect. One version (designated "A") was recorded in standard English. The second version (designated "B") was spoken in Black English. The author, who is bidialectal, spoke both versions. Two white female graduate students separately went to various public locations in a southwestern community and asked people if they would mind participating in a survey. Upon their consent, each participant listened to both versions of the tape and afterward, were asked the following questions:

1. Which speaker, in your opinion, might be the smarter one?
2. Which speaker would you most enjoy talking with and why?

3. Which speaker talks better?
4. a. What kind of job would "A" have?
   b. What kind of job would "B" have?
   c. Which one would you hire?
5. Which speaker would you rather
   a. Be your teacher (This was asked to the children.)
   b. Teach your children (This was asked to the adults.)

A total of twenty people participated in this project. The responses to the first question are summarized in Table 6-I.

As can be seen, the majority of people chose the standard English speaker as the smarter one (14 people) while the remainder of the participants were either uncommitted or considered both speakers to be equally smart. No respondent indicated that speaker B was smarter. All but one of the black participants judged speaker A as the smarter one.

A little more than half of the participants (11 persons) responded that they would most enjoy talking with the standard English speaker (Table 6-II). Three people would enjoy talking with speaker B more; six people would enjoy talking with either speaker, both speakers, or were uncommitted. Three people did respond that they would enjoy talking with speaker B more. However, the participants' responses still seemed to reflect essentially negative views toward speaker B's speech regardless of choice of speaker. Most participants who would prefer talking with speaker A indicated that speaker A would be clearer and easier to understand. One participant would prefer talking with speaker B because this speaker was presumed to have a "more colorful personality."

All 20 participants, regardless of age, race, gender, or occupation selected the standard English speaker as the better speaker (Table 6-III). Participants' reasons for this choice were similar: the standard English speaker used better, clearer speech. Even a black high school student stated that speaker B's "speech is not proper." It is interesting to note that some of the participants responded with dialectal variations similar to those of speaker B and seemed to be unaware of these non-standard patterns in their own speech.

Responses to the questions concerning jobs speakers A and B were presumed to have are summarized in Table 6-IV. Although teacher, writer, store worker, secretary, and researcher* were

---

*The participant who responded "researcher" for both speakers became aware of the study.

Cultural Language Differences

Table 6-I

LISTENERS' JUDGEMENTS REGARDING
SPEAKER WHO IS SMARTER

Age (years)	Race	Sex	Occupation	Which Speaker in your opinion, might be the smarter one?
7	Wh	F		A
7	Wh	M		A
9	Wh	F		A
9	Bl	F		A
10	Wh	M		A
12	Wh	M		A
12	Wh	M		A
12	Bl	M		A
15	Wh	M	High School	both probably smart; if B's an old lady, she's probably not smart
16	Bl	M	High School	A
19	Wh	F		can't tell just by listening
21	Wh	F	Student	A
22	Wh	F	Student	A
23	Wh	F	Student	A
29	Bl	M		both on same level
	Wh	M	Jr. Hi. History Teacher	Uncommitted
	Wh	M	College Professor	Uncommitted
	Wh	F	Unemployed (college degree)	Uncommitted
	Wh	F	Housewife (college degree)	A
	Wh	M	Pilot (college degree)	A

A = Standard English Speaker
B = Black English Speaker

Table 6-II

LISTENERS' PREFERENCE FOR SPEAKER THEY
WOULD MOST ENJOY TALKING WITH

Age (years)	Race	Sex	Occupation	Which Speaker Would You Most Enjoy Talking With?	Why?
7	Wh	F		A	
7	Wh	M		A	
9	Wh	F		A	
9	Bl	F		Uncommitted	
10	Wh	M		A	Probably understand 'em better
12	Wh	M		A	It'd be easier to understand A; couldn't understand B very much
12	Wh	M		A	Can understand 'em more better
12	Bl	M		B	
15	Wh	M	High School	A	B sounds like an old lady
16	Bl	M	High School	A	Can understand it better
19	Wh	F		Either	
21	Wh	F	Student	A	
22	Wh	F	Student	Either	
23	Wh	F	Student	A	More clearer to listener
29	Bl	M		Both	Both seem to be informative
	Wh	M	Jr. Hi. History Teacher	Uncommitted	
	Wh	M	College Professor	A	
	Wh	F	Unemployed (college degree)	B	
	Wh	F	Housewife (college degree)	B	More colorful personality
	Wh	M	Pilot . (college degree)	Uncommitted	

= Standard English Speaker
= Black English Speaker

Cultural Language Differences

Table 6-III

LISTENERS' JUDGMENTS REGARDING THE
SPEAKER WHO TALKS BETTER

Age (years)	Race	Sex	Occupation	Which Speaker Talks Best?	Why?
7	Wh	F		A	
7	Wh	M		A	
9	Wh	F		A	
9	Bl	F		A	
10	Wh	M		A	B's leavin' words out
12	Wh	M		A	More plain and clear
12	Wh	M		A	B's kinda blurry
12	Bl	M		A	
15	Wh	M	High School	A	Clearer; just talks better
16	Bl	M	High School	A	B's speech is not proper
19	Wh	F		A	Clearer
21	Wh	F	Student	A	
22	Wh	F	Student	A	Talks more standard
23	Wh	F	Student	A	Better English
29	Bl	M		A	A lot more clarity
	Wh	M	Jr. Hi. History Teacher	A	
	Wh	M	College Professor	A	╲
	Wh	F	Unemployed (college degree)	A	
	Wh	F	Housewife (college degree)	A	
	Wh	M	Pilot (college degree)	A	

A = Standard English Speaker
B = Black English Speaker

Table 6-IV

LISTENERS' INFERENCES OF OCCUPATIONS HELD BY STANDARD ENGLISH (A) AND BLACK ENGLISH (B) SPEAKERS

Age (years)	Race	Sex	Occupation	Job Would A Have?	Job Would B Have?	Would You Have?
7	Wh	F		Works at grocery		
7	Wh	M				
9	Wh	F				
9	Bl	F				
10	Wh	M			Probably a maid	
12	Wh	M		Teacher	She wouldn't have a very good job 'cause they would think she wasn't very smart	
12	Wh	M		Writer	Writer	
12	Bl	M				
15	Wh	M	High School	Works in a store	Retired	
16	Bl	M	High School	Secretary	Works in a store	
19	Wh	F		Secretary	Teaching	
21	Wh	F	Student			A
22	Wh	F	Student	Teacher	Secretary	
23	Wh	F	Student	Teacher	Maid	
29	Bl	M		Researcher	Researcher	
	Wh	M	Jr. Hi. History Teacher			Uncommitted
	Wh	M	College Professor			A
	Wh	F	Unemployed (college degree)			A
	Wh	F	Housewife (college degree)			A
	Wh	M	Pilot (college degree)			A

　　　　　　　Cultural Language Differences

Table 6-V

LISTENERS' PREFERENCES FOR THE STANDARD ENGLISH (A) OR BLACK ENGLISH (B) AS A TEACHER

Age (years)	Race	Sex	Occupation	Which Speaker Would you Rather. . .	
				Be Your Teacher?	Teach your Children?
7	Wh	M		A	
9	Wh	F		A	
9	Bl	F		Uncommitted	
12	Bl	M		Uncommitted	
21	Wh	F	Student	Uncommitted	A
	Wh	M	Jr. Hi. History Teacher		A
	Wh	M	College Professor		A
	Wh	F	Unemployed (college degree)		A
	Wh	F	Housewife (college degree)		A
	Wh	M	Pilot (college degree)		A

offered as occupations for both speakers, two participants thought the dialect speaker to be a maid and one participant stated that the dialect speaker "wouldn't have a very good job." None of these responses were offered as occupations for the standard English speaker. Additionally, with the exception of one uncommitted response, participants who were asked which speaker they would hire selected the standard English speaker.

Finally, responses to teacher preference are summarized in Table 6-V. The two black children were uncommitted in their choice of a teacher. However, the white children chose the standard English speaker as the one they would prefer. Additionally, the adults who were asked which speaker they would prefer to teach their children chose the standard English speaker.

It is stressed that the results just reported are from a pilot study that was designed to determine if layperson bias should receive research attention at all and to determine the best possible methodology for investigating this question. Among other things, the pilot study was limited in size of sample, question format (i.e., forced-choice), and manner of questioning (i.e., not all participants were given the opportunity to respond to all of the questions). As a result, valid conclusions cannot be reached on the basis of the pilot study results alone. However, when taken collectively with the result of previous literature, these results do suggest that layperson bias is a problem that deserves our further exploration.

Since there is only rudimentary evidence to substantiate the existence of layperson bias, then it follows that even less attention has been paid to examining why society reacts differentially to dialect speakers and to other physical and cultural factors that are associated with various minority groups. It is speculated that layperson bias toward dialect speakers probably is a result of dialect origin. According to Burling (1973), a major hypothesis to explain the origin of dialects is that whenever social groups are divided, their dialects diverge.

Using Black English as an example of how this hypothesis might account for current societal attitudes, the separation of blacks from whites in the United States has been a major source of dialect divergence. The earliest beginnings of the dialect was Pidgin, which was a simplified, reduced form of English. Pidgin was used between Europeans and Africans because of the necessity to immediately communicate basic wants and needs. However, since both races knew there would never be an intimate contact between them to form a unified speech community, the Africans had no consistent or reliable source of English to imitate. Additionally, the African slaves needed a common means of communication between themselves since African slaves came from a number of African communities which spoke a variety of languages. As a result, Pidgin English began to include many African words and as it became an everyday language, it evolved into a creole. Due to the continued separation of the races and the progression of the dialect through generations, Black English has evolved into its present form. Various morphological structures (such as multiple negation), vocabulary items, and tonal qualities of Black English can be traced to the characteristics of certain African languages. During slavery, blacks were not only "encouraged" to use the dialect, but also were subject to punishment for attempting to "sound white." Speech patterns used by whites were equated with reading and writing ability, mathematical skill, financial/social status, and political power. All of these were generally denied to the black slave. As a result, the dialect currently spoken by many black people, although rich in heritage, is probably still associated with lack of educational achievement among blacks in the perceptions of the public. The historical association between being black and being uneducated could also explain why minority professionals may be initially presumed to be less capable than non-minority clinical service providers.

Some empirical evidence suggests that at least one reason to explain why the layperson may react differentially toward the professional who chooses to serve economically disadvantaged and minority groups is cultural mistrust (Terrell and Terrell, 1981). Cultural mistrust is a term used to explain the level of suspiciousness black individuals have for whites. To measure this level of suspiciousness, an Inventory to Measure Cultural Mistrust among Blacks (CMI) was developed for black adults (Terrell and Terrell, 1981) and a second CMI for black children, (Terrell, Terrell, and Flint, 1982). Follow-up studies utilizing the scales indicate that black adults and children who have a high level of cultural mistrust tend to perform more poorly on an intelligence test when the test is administered by a white examiner than when it is given by a black examiner (Terrell, Terrell and Taylor, 1981; Terrell and Terrell, 1983). An additional study suggests that level of cultural mistrust may influence premature termination from psychological counseling services (Terrell and Terrell, 1983b). These authors' findings indicate that blacks with high cultural mistrust levels are more likely to discontinue from counseling prematurely when assigned to a white counselor than when assigned to a black counselor. Even though these studies were designed to measure and investigate the implications of cultural mistrust among blacks, these findings may have applicability to understanding the biases that may occur when any low income or minority group receives clinical services from a professional who is not a member of that group.

In summary, only scant literature exists to substantiate the current presence of layperson bias and the types of bias that can occur. Why the public reacts differentially to dialect speakers, minority professionals, and the professionals who serve disadvantaged and minority groups, can only be speculated at this time due to the lack of empirical evidence. However, it may be that accounts of dialect origin and evolution can serve as interim, partial explanations for society's reactions toward dialect speakers and minority speech and language professionals. Additionally, layperson and client mistrust of the clinician who is not a member of the layperson's or client's ethnic group may be one explanation for layperson bias toward nonminority professionals who provide clinical services to minority individuals.

PERSONAL ACCOUNTS OF TYPES OF LAYPERSON BIAS

Marsha, a white speech-language pathologist, related her experiences with various biases during a tape-recorded interview conducted in 1983. Marsha has been providing speech pathology services for the past four years to Miller Middle School, which is located in a southwestern geographic area. The school has a predominately black student body and is situated in a black, low-income community. Prior to this current position, Marsha provided diagnostic and therapy services to a school located in the West. The students who attended this school were of many racial and ethnic backgrounds. During the interview, Marsha stated that she had no hesitation about working with any child, regardless of background. She thoroughly enjoys her current position and desires to continue at Miller School.

The black speech-language pathologist, who will be referred to as Lynn in this paper, contributed her recollections in writing instead of by cassette tape. After receiving her Master's degree in speech pathology from a northern university, Lynn relocated to a southern state and provided services to two rural elementary schools in 1974-75, just several years after these schools had been desegregated. At that time, Lynn was the only black speech-language pathologist in the district's school system. Lynn held that employment position for one year. Since that time, Lynn has relocated to a southwestern area where she supervises speech-language pathology students in a university training program.

Proper names of people and schools have been changed. General geographic areas have been substituted for the names of specific states.

Layperson Bias Toward Dialect Speakers
Experiences

The following excerpts from Marsha and Lynn's anecdotes illustrate different ways in which laypersons may react toward dialect speakers and various minorities.

Marsha: "When I told people that I would be coming here, that I would be moving to the Southwest, they asked me what I would be doing. Will you teach? and I said well, yes, I'll be a speech therapist just like I've always been and the remarks made to me were 'well how are you gunna tell whether those people in the Southwest have an accent or not, and how will you tell if they've got a bona fide speech problem? And the whole prejudice tended toward southern speakers, not just one particular minority group over another, but just southern speakers in general. I remember one person said to me 'well those people don't have any "r's," they don't say any "r's." Are you going to teach them their "r's"? 'I really don't know what I'm going to do. I'm going to wait 'till I get there and see what I'm going to do.' So that was one incident. Well, it represents a kind of stereotype that regions may have toward another regional area and also a lack of understanding or education about standard English or standard regional English."

"My school assignment to Miller was four years ago; this is my fourth year and at the time I was assigned there the only part of this school that was integrated was the staff, and the whole Miller area which involved three schools, elementary, middle, and high school were all black in an all-black community except for one or two white families, and I had no problems about going and working in the area at all. I'd worked with multi-racial faculties and kids before. It was not anything I gave any thought to. Other people in the area or in my community made remarks you know, like 'well, you'll have to scale down your goals for the students.' And I kind of sloughed that off and said 'well, it depends on what the levels are of the students I'll be working with,' and that's true of any school anywhere. Most of the remarks came from people who were not familiar with education and who had never taught, never been around other people other than their own little set group. Other professionals made no remarks to me. Some people said that it would be a difficult neighborhood to work in or a difficult community to drive in . I've found that totally untrue.

"I do remember when I was working in an elementary school, and it was a mixed school, we had a resource teacher who invariably (in staffings), whenever a black student was discussed as to whether or not this child would work out all right in regular classes in middle school, would ask where that child was going to middle school and if the kid was going to Miller she'd say, 'well it doesn't matter then. He'll fit right in with the rest of them' which I found to be a particularly offensive remark to make. But I didn't have any experience or knowledge or anything to put her down, to tell her she didn't know what she was talking about. Whenever we get a very low child in the middle school who should have been shuttled to a special school from elementary, he still belongs in a special school regardless. Now if I were back in that situation with that particular person again I might open my mouth. This was two years prior to my being assigned to Miller, so it really hasn't been long. But her particular attitude toward dialect speakers or black kids, I'll speak quite frankly because that's what we've been talking about, her attitude, I thought, was totally irresponsible and unprofessional, and yet I had no experience and nothing to back up my attitudes or my feelings about her. I hadn't ever been at Miller so I didn't know who was there, I didn't know what the staff was like. For all I knew, she was speaking the truth. Somehow I thought she was probably not, but (I thought) surely that woman is not that naive. But I do remember that particular incident because it comes back to me frequently. We still get students from that school who need to have been referred to special schools but were placed in regular classes in middle school with resource help and they're floundering because they were misplaced and I know it's because she's still making this remark. She just has to be or else we wouldn't be getting these kids. I haven't spoken with the speech therapist at that school to know if that's still going on.

"Sometimes, people will ask me questions about 'well, do you have to scale down your objectives or how do you deal with the kids who speak black English,' and I tell them, 'I just say "hi" to them in the halls and go about my business.' What else can I do?, I say "hi" to them just like I do any other kid. What's to deal with? But I think remarks like that come mainly out of ignorance and a lack of experience maybe with Black English speakers. I know that there are some people who choose not to acknowledge other people, but in most people, it's probably just a lack of experience of getting to know other people."

Lynn: "At Abrams School, all the kids were given an IQ test at the beginning of the school year and on the basis of what a kid's score was, that kid was put into regular classes, or classes for the gifted, emotionally disturbed, specific learning disabled, reading, or educable mentally retarded. The mentally retarded classroom was self-contained and it was hard for me to figure out why one little rural school would need all those special programs. And then there was me, the speech pathologist. I guess what was most disturbing to me was that there was no recognition of cultural differences or the fact that many of those kids at Abrams were economically disavantaged. I am convinced that some of the kids in the mentally retarded class weren't mentally retarded at all. I remember one little girl that came to me for therapy. Her name was Billie Joe. She was twelve years old, black, and in the educable mentally retarded classroom. I became very good friends with her teacher in this MR class and we often talked with each other about the kids that both of us taught. Anyway, this teacher felt that Billie Joe was really trainable mentally retarded, and should be in that kind of class except that the school did not have one. I can't remember exactly how it came about, but I began to make plans to take Billie Joe home with me for a weekend. Billie Joe's mother packed a few of her daughter's clothes, which smelled of urine, signed the permission slip with her "X," and Billie Joe and I headed for my home. We stopped off at a discount store in town and I helped Billie Joe pick out a few short sets, underwear, and shoes. We were waiting in a rather long check-out line, and Billie Joe was moving back and forth holding her things, when she said, "Miz Jones, we can get out faster in the line down there" and off she went with me trailing behind her. And we did get out faster in that line. I remember thinking, this kid is supposed to be trainable mentally retarded and I was the one who felt stupid because I didn't see that another line was moving more quickly. Another time that weekend, I asked Billie Joe what she would like for me to do about something, I don't remember exactly what it was, but I do remember her answer which was "It's your house, Miz Jones." I also found out that this kid was very mannerly but had a street wisdom beyond her years. She knew about sex, knew where babies came from, and had a sense of the value of money. Does this sound like a mentally retarded kid? Anyway, I told Billie Joe's teacher about what I thought about Billie Joe. Needless to say, my insights were definitely not appreciated. Who was I to tell her who was or wasn't mentally retarded, Billie Joe was not only mentally retarded, but so was her whole family and they ought to be sterilized so they don't keep having mentally retarded kids. She broke off our friendship after that. But I didn't mind that so much as I felt powerless to help Billie Joe and the other kids that were also labeled and put in special classes where they shouldn't have been. I think it was around that point that I decided to work in a university where I could tell students about such biases before they get out on their own. I never could figure out why Billie Joe's teacher reacted the way she did. She was black too so it couldn't have been a racial issue. The only other reason I could think of is that I stepped into her boundary of expertise. It could have been a financial thing too. If someone went around identifying the kids in her class who weren't mentally retarded, they'd identify her right out of her job. After all this time, I still wonder about how Billie Joe is doing and wonder if things have changed any at that school in seven years."

Discussion

The personal experiences of these two professionals illustrate two different reactions laypersons may have toward dialect speakers or toward various poor, minority individuals. First, reactions were made toward the speech patterns of regional dialect speakers. According to Marsha's experience, people of one geographic region view speakers of another regional dialect as having speech patterns that merit remediation in a speech therapy program. Although regional and social dialects are currently accepted as legitimate linguistic variations of English among speech and language professionals, the public may still ascribe to the deficiency view, due to a lack of accurate information about these speech patterns.

Second, both speech-language pathologists experienced situations in which laypersons, who in these cases were educators, made erroneous judgments about the abilities of black children based upon biased test results and lack of other information. In Marsha's anecdote, black children were denied appropriate special help in a predominately black middle school because of a referring teacher's assumption that all the black students who attended that school had depressed academic performance. In Lynn's experience, poor and minority children were inappropriately classified as mentally retarded based upon test results that did not account for the cultural and economic background of the children. This was also the type of bias with which both professionals felt powerless to effect change. This may have been due to the fact that neither speech-language pathologist had the authority to change the situation or to even ask for justification regarding placement decisions for individual low income, minority children.

Layperson Bias Toward Professionals Who Choose to Serve Dialect Speakers:

Experiences

The following excerpt from Marsha's experiences illustrate two kinds of reactions laypersons may have toward speech-language pathologists who primarily provide clinical services within low-income, dialect speaking communities.

Marsha: "I really haven't run into too many problems or incidents with students or the faculty. I did have one kid ask me why I was teaching him to talk like a honky and I fell out on the floor laughing. I just sat there and looked for a while and finally I just started gigling. . . I couldn't help it, it was so funny. He just kind of looked, finally he got embarrassed and he just looked away and we never did discuss it any more. After that I guess he finally realized the ridiculousness of what he said. And I said to him, he had a black speech therapist earlier sometime along the way, and I said 'didn't she require the same things of you that I'm requiring?' Well, he said 'yes,' and I said, 'well, let's go on and do our work. We've had enough of this.'"

"Sometimes I have people make or ask curious questions, you know, like 'how do you like it *there*?' meaning MIller, like it's another world you're going to. And I always say, 'well, I asked to be returned, so I must like it.'"

Discussion

This excerpt illustrates two ways in which a speech-language pathologist who serves minority individuals may encounter biased reactions. First, the minority client/patient may question the motives of the speech-language pathologist who is not a member of the client/patient's racial or ethnic group. This may be due to the minority individual's cultural mistrust or suspiciousness of the non-minority professional, as it has been discussed earlier in this paper. The fact that the child asked Marsha about her motives allowed her to resolve the situation. However, it is possible that there are minority individuals who would never openly ask a non-minority professional about his/her intentions. In these cases, the non-minority speech-language pathologist may come under close scrutiny over a period of time until he/she checks out as someone who can be trusted.

Another kind of bias illustrated in this excerpt may be the perception by laypersons that professionals who provide services primarily to low income and various minority groups are less fortunate than professionals who serve affluent individuals. This bias rings of an "oh, you poor thing" reaction, and the lack of understanding on the part of laypersons why any professional would enjoy working in a position where a disproportionate amount of the caseload consists of poor, minority individuals.

Layperson Bias Toward Minority Professionals:

Experiences

In the following excerpt, Lynn relates her experience with a biased reaction from a parent.

Lynn: "When I was at Abrams, I didn't have any incidents with prejudice that I can recall with the faculty and students. The biggest problem I had with them was lack of understanding about what a speech-language pathologist does. The faculty called me "speech teacher" and some of the kids called me "speech lady." But it was some of the parents I really had problems with . I remember one incident. After I had finished all my screening, I was setting up my caseload when one of the parents called on the phone to make sure that her daughter would be enrolled in therapy. The little girl, I'll call her Cathy, was white and she had a severe articulation problem. I assured the mother that Cathy would be enrolled and suggested that we meet to discuss therapy goals for the year and to get the permission forms signed. Of course, I spoke to her in standard English as I always do when I'm working even though I also speak Black

English. At the set day and time, Cathy's mother arrived at the school and when I came out to the lobby to meet her, her eyes widened and her bottom lip dropped. She came back to my room and the conference went along very well. Cathy did make good progress in therapy. At the next conference with Cathy's mother, I think it was at the end of the year, the visit again went very well. As I walked her to the lobby she said 'Oh, I just wanted to let you know, after the last time we met, I went home and told Cathy's grandmother that you was colored. And she said how in the world was a negra gonna teach Cathy how to talk, but I told her you talk just fine and you do just as good as the last speech teacher Cathy had.' I suppose that remark could have really offended me, and it did to some extent. The sorry part about the whole thing was this adding up process, that is 'if you're black, you speak a dialect; if you speak a dialect, then you're not competent; and if you're black, you're not competent until you prove that you are.' What made it so bad is that the kid's mother thought I would be so pleased with this "complement." I know that I responded to her remarks by saying something like, "Thank you so much. I am so pleased that Cathy has made so much progress this year." But I just knew that she had waited all that year to make up her mind whether or not I was competent to treat her daughter's speech problems."

Discussion

Lynn's experience illustrates several views laypersons may have toward minority speech and language professionals. Based upon Lynn's experience, there may be the assumption that all minorities use speech patterns characteristic of their ethnic or racial group. Many black people do not use dialect. Neither can the assumption be made that everyone of Hispanic background speaks Spanish.

A second, and perhaps more important bias that Lynn encountered was the assumption that a minority speech-language pathologist is less competent than a non-minority professional. The historical relationship between minorities, dialect, and lack of educational opportunity as discussed earlier in this paper is a possible explanation for this view. For this reason, Cathy's family may have assumed that Lynn's professional training was substandard. The family may have also believed that Lynn's professional competence did not (or should not) extend to providing clinical services to middle-class white children.

MANAGEMENT PRINCIPLES

As it has been previously stated, there is a paucity of evidence which acknowledges the presence of layperson bias. It is therefore understandable why no literature exists that proposes how negative public reactions toward dialect speakers, minority professionals, and professionals who work with dialect speakers might be best resolved. Since there may be a number of speech and language specialists who presently encounter such biases, it seems necessary to propose some immediate general principles for layperson bias management that can be used until research into this area is generated.

The two speech-language pathologists who shared their personal experiences earlier in this paper had similar insights and ways of handling their individual incidences of societal bias. The following layperson bias management principles are primarily based upon these similarities. The principles are therefore simple and more common-sense than scholarly.

1. *Assume that a biased remark or behavior is primarily due to an individual society member's lack of knowledge about other groups of people.*

This principle does not deny the existence of deeply engrained bigotry toward various dialect-speaking and minority groups. More than likely there are no general management principles that can affect attitude change in such individuals. However, this principle does give the speech and language professional a basis for teaching and sharing factual information about dialect-speaking groups with uninformed members of society. The shared information may not result in a change in the society member's biased attitudes. At the very least, however, the society member's increased awareness may minimize the reoccurrence of biased reactions in the presence of the speech and language professional who provided the information.

2. *Be thoroughly informed of dialectal characteristics and relevant literature.*

Prior to any attempt to share sociolinguistic information with members of the public, it is incumbent that a thorough current knowledge of sociolinguistic literature, normal dialectal patterns of the minority group being served, and nondiscriminatory assessment techniques be obtained. The professional will have difficulty sharing information that he/she does not clearly understand.

3. *Take the path of least resistance.* *

This principle does not imply that speech and language professionals should compromise their stance regarding the cultural difference view. This principle merely recognizes that 1) management tactics will vary, depending upon the status of the individual who performed the biased reaction, and 2) these tactics should result in minimal damage to the dialect-speaking patient/student and to the speech and language professional.

For example, the path of least resistance for a minority speech-language pathologist who receives a biased remark from a non-minority parent (see Lynn's previous anecdote) is to react politely, but continue to perform assignments in a professional manner. The path of least resistance for managing biased remarks made by a belligerent dinner guest may be to state firm objections to the remarks and then simply walk away or leave. As another example, consider a public school speech-language pathologist whose supervisor places minority children in inappropriate classrooms on the basis of test scores and other partial, stereotyped information. The path of least resistance for this situation may be to suggest to the supervisor that an inservice in the area of nondiscriminatory assessment would be an interesting and helpful topic for everyone. An expert with no affiliation with the school could be invited to conduct the inservice. Of course, the principal would be in attendance.

If the path of least resistance is not followed in each of these examples, the result may be more harm than good. In the first example, confronting the parent in a face-to-face exchange of emotion may result in interrupted services to the children if the professional is terminated from her position. In the second example, the professional could possibly risk physical harm in a fight. If a least resistant path is not followed, in the third example, (i.e. use of a more direct approach to confront the supervisor's biases), it is likely that the supervisor may take offense and service delivery to the minority children would not be improved.

An attempt has been made to propose some general management principles that have applicability to various types of layperson bias. However, since the principles were based upon the experiences of only two speech-language pathologists, it is not known to what ex-

---

*Contributed by "Marsha" during taped interview.

tent these guidelines can be applied to situations that differ from those experiences. Additionally, it is not known whether the principles can even be used to manage situations that appear similar to the experiences of the two professionals. Such similar-appearing incidents may actually contain some unidentified factors that could influence a principle's effectiveness. For example, it is questionable whether a non-minority parent would be willing to consider a minority speech-language pathologist to be a competent professional if the parent does not observe significant improvement in his/her child's speech and language skills. Therefore, the proposed layperson bias management principles should be used with caution, pending empirical investigation of this area.

CONCLUSION

Based upon existing evidence, we can conclude with reasonable certainty that layperson bias toward dialect speakers and toward professionals who provide services to dialect speakers does exist. Furthermore, there is evidence that layperson bias toward minority language specialists also occurs. However, there is no literature available to explain exactly what these biases are nor how they can best be managed. This paper attempted to identify several types of layperson bias by relating the experiences of two speech-language pathologists. The paper also discussed how these biases might be resolved.

Due to the paucity of research on this topic, conclusions regarding the problems and solutions of layperon bias illustrated in this paper must contain some caveats. First, one should not assume that layperson bias only occurs between blacks and whites and only in Southern geographic areas. Southern black and white participants were used as examples in this paper only because these were the only people contacted who agreed to contribute their experiences. (A Hispanic speech-language pathologist also consented via telephone conversation, but the requested antedote was never received.) However, it is highly likely that layperson bias does occur among other racial, ethnic, and regional groups. For example, it is probable that the white language professional from a middle-class background who provides clinical services to an isolated Appalachian dialect-speaking community may experience layperson bias due to being an "outsider." The clinician who encounters mistrust of her professional activities among Native American people and the parent who complains that a Hispanic-American speech-language pathologist should not provide therapy services for her child because of an "accent" which really does not exist are also probable examples of layperson bias.

Another caution is that it is not known to what extent the problems and solutions of the two professionals presented in this paper are representative of the experiences of bias among other speech-language pathologists. There is also no indication as to which biases occur more frequently than the others, or which ones are now less problematic than they were five to seven years ago. Furthermore, there may be additional types of layperson bias that have not been discussed here because they have not yet been identified.

Finally, the focus of this paper does not imply that biases no longer exist among speech-language pathologists. Marsha related an incident that occurred during a meeting of her colleagues at the beginning of the school year. When Marsha told the others that she had been assigned to Miller School, one of these colleagues remarked "I'm glad it wasn't me." Marsha has also been asked by a colleague whether "they" (i.e. the students at Miller) have "torn up" the new Miller school building yet. Indeed, there is still a need for speech and language professionals to continue to educate one another and to share information regarding dialects and minority issues. However, a major point of this paper is that this information must also be shared with the public.

Perhaps more than anything else, the background literature, personal experiences, and management principles discussed in this paper have attempted to provide evidence that layperson bias is an issue worthy of our attention. Much previous research and writing efforts have been directed toward demonstrating *to language specialists* that social dialects and the persons who use them should not be viewed as deficient. However, the same zeal by which we undertook the task of educating and convincing each other on non-discriminatory views has not been applied in a large-scale effort toward educating the public of this stance. As a result, negative attitudes toward dialect systems and toward various poor and minority groups who traditionally use dialects continue to prevail among the public. Within various educational, employment, and social situations, dialect speakers continue to be viewed by laypersons as communicatively handicapped in direct contrast to nondiscriminatory assessment and treatment programs. The difference view is of little avail if society will not allow dialect speaking and minority individuals to realize the benefits of nonbiased clinical services. Research designed to document, identify, and provide strategies for the management of layperson biases is long overdue.

Appendix

STANDARD ENGLISH VERSION

Hi! How are you on this hot day? I am talking to you through this tape because I have suggestions for you on how to stay cool in hot weather such as this. First, wear white or light colored clothing. Second, use a wide brimmed hat to keep the sun out of your eyes. Third, eat light meals and drink drinks that do not have sugar in them. These are just a few but time doesn't permit me to give you any more. I hope you are able to keep your cool until winter comes. Thank you for listening. Good bye!

BLACK ENGLISH VERSION

Hey! How you doin' on dis here hot day? I be talkin' to you through dis here tape 'cause I hab' questions fo' you on how ta stay coo' in such hot weather such as dis' here. Firs', wear white or light color clothes. Secon', use a wide-brim hat ta keep da sun outta yo' eyes. Third, eat light meals and drink drinks which ain't got no sugar in dem'. Dese is jus' a few, but time don't permit me ta give you no mo'. I hope you be able ta keep yo' coo' 'til winter come. Thank you fo' lis'nin'. Goo'bye!

REFERENCES

Baratz, J.C. A Bi-dialectal Task for Determining Language Proficiency in Economically Disadvantaged Negro Children. *Child Development*, 1969, *40*, 889-901.

Baratz, J.C. and Shuy, R.W. (Eds.). *Teaching Black Children to Read.* Washington, D.C.: Center for Applied Linguistics, 1969.

Bereiter, C. and Engelmann, S. *Teaching Disadvantaged Children in the Preschool.* Englewood Cliffs, N.J.: Prentice-Hall, 1966.

Burling, R. *English in Black and White.* New York: Holt, Rinehart and Winston, 1975.

Butler, K.G. and Terrell, S.L. (Eds.). Non-biased Assessment of Language Differences. *Topics in Language Disorders,* 1983, *3.*

Deutsch, M. The Roll of Social Class in Language Development and Cognition. *American Journal of Orthopsychiatry,* 1965, *25,* 78-88.

Felice, L.W. Black Student Dropout Behavior: Disengagement from School Rejection and Racial Discrimination. *Journal of Negro Education,* 1981, *20,* 415-525.

Holland, A.L. Nonbiased Assessment and Treatment of Adults who Have Neurologic Speech and Language Problems. *Topics in Language Disorders,* 1983, *3,* 67-75.

Houston, S.H. A Re-examination of Some Assumptions About the Language of the Disadvantaged Child. *Child Development,* 1970, *41,* 947-963.

John, V. The Intellectual Development of Slum Children: Some Preliminary Findings. *American Journal of Orthopsychiatry,* 1963, *33,* 813-822.

Kochman, T. *Rappin and Stylin out in the Black Community.* Champaign: University of Illinois Press, 1971.

Kutner, B., Wilkins, C., and Yarrow, P.R. Verbal Attitudes and Overt Behavior Involving Racial Prejudice. *Journal of Abnormal and Clinical Psychology,* 1952, *47,* 649-652.

Labov, W. *The Social Stratification of English in New York City.* Washington, D.C.: Center for Applied Linguistics, 1966.

Osser, H., Wang, M.D., and Zaid, F. The Young Child's Ability to Imitate and Comprehend Speech: A Comparison of Two Subcultural Groups. *Child Development,* 1969, *40,* 1063-1075.

Rosenthal, M. The Magic Boxes: Preschool Children's Attitudes Toward Black and Standard English. *The Florida FL Reporter,* 1974, *12,* 55-62.

Shuy, R.W. A Linguistic Background for Developing Beginning Reading Materials for Black Children. In J.C. Baratz and R.W. Shuy (Eds.), *Teaching Black Children to Read.* Washington, D.C.: Center for Applied Linguistics, 1969.

Social Dialects: Position Paper. Prepared by Committee on Status of Racial Minorities, American Speech-Language-Hearing Association. *Asha,* 1983, *25,* 23-24.

Seymour, H. and Miller-Jones, D. Language and Cognitive Assessment of Black Children. *Speech and Language: Advances in Basic Research and Practice.* New York: Academic Press, 1981.

Taylor, O.L. Language Differences. In G.H. Shames and E.H. Wiig (Eds.), *Human Communication Disorders, An Introduction.* Columbus, Ohio: Merrill, 1982.

Terrell, F. Dialectal Differences Between Middle Class Black and White Children Who Do and Do Not Associate With Lower Class Black Children. *Language and Speech,* 1975, *18,* 65-73.

Terrell, F. and Miller, F.S. The Development of an Inventory to Measure Experience with Racialistic Incidents Among Blacks. Unpublished manuscript, Texas Christian University, 1980.

Terrell, F. and Terrell, S.L. An Inventory to Measure Cultural Mistrust Among Blacks. *The Western Journal of Black Studies,* 1981, *5,* 180-185.

Terrell, F. And Terrell, S.L., and Golin, S. Language Productivity of Black and White Children in Black Versus White Situations. *Language and Speech,* 1977, *20,* 377-383.

Terrell, F. and Terrell, S.L. Race of Counselor, Cultural Mistrust Level, and Premature Termination From Counseling Among Black Clients. Unpublished manuscript, 1983.

Terrell, F. and Terrell, S.L. The Relationship Between Race of Examiner, Cultural Mistrust, and the Intelligence Test Performance of Black Children. *Psychology in the Schools,* 1983, *20,* 367-369.

Terrell, F., Terrell, S.L., and Flint, L. Development of an inventory to Measure Cultural Mistrust in Black Children. Paper presented at the 15th annual convention of the Association of Black Psychologists, Cincinnati, 1982.

Terrell, F., Terrell, S.L., and Taylor, J. Effects of Race of Examiner and Cultural Mistrust on the WAIS Performance of Black Students. *Journal of Consulting and Clinical Psychology,* 1981, *49,* 750-751.

Terrell, S.L. Attitudes toward Black and Standard English Speakers. Unpublished manuscript, North Texas State University, 1981.

Terrell, S.L. and Terrell, F. Effects of Speaking Black English Upon Employment Opportunities. *Asha,* 1983, *25,* 27-29.

Williams, R. And Wolfram, W. *Social Dialects: Differences Versus Disorders.* Rockville, Md.: American Speech-Language-Hearing Association, 1977.

Williams, R.L. An Afrocentric Approach to the Assessment of Blacks. Guest lecture presented to the Department of Psychology, North Texas State University, March, 1981.

Chapter VII

LANGUAGE INTERVENTION IN THE SCHOOL AND IN THE CLINIC:

The Role of the Speech-Language Pathologist in School and Non-school Environments

BETHEL H. WOMACK

INTRODUCTION

I N 1970, Venezky (1970) noted that the child whose linguistic skills differ markedly from the socially acceptable standard of the school system faces overt and covert discrimination in education. Furthermore, on the interpersonal level the classroom peers view this child as peculiar. The child is perceived as being inferior. The teacher may not understand everything this child says and might have difficulty viewing non-standard dialect as being anything other than a substandard speech pattern. We doubt there has been much change in the classroom throughout the country in this day and time. The reading programs are not equipped for such dialect speaking children. Readiness tests, reading materials, and teacher guides with rare exceptions are designed solely for middle-class standard English speakers. For non-standard dialect speaking children there is no readily available guide which distinguishes dialect differences from standard English, or suggests how academic subjects could be effectively taught to such children. As Venezky pointed out then or now, non-standard English speakers do not fit comfortably into existing school systems.

As Adler emphasizes elsewhere in this book, there are three major issues involved with non-standard English speakers. First, there is a significant interrelationship between talking and reading/ writing skill development, i.e., the attainment of literacy; because of this relationship some speakers of social dialect often manifest poor academic skills. Second, the public's negative stereotypic perception of social dialect speakers cause many otherwise competent adults to have difficulty finding work appropriate to their skills. Third, there is a need for such a speaker to learn to talk in standard or establishment English, but strategies used to teach establishment English have generally been ineffective.

How to obviate these problems is the focus of this chapter. In particular, the speech-language pathologist's role is of critical importance. Necessary skills for the speech-language pathologist will be addressed in the following pages.

Language and Education

The development of language is basic to the expression and enhancement of intelligence. It takes approximately 10 years for a child to develop adult language. By age five, a child's speech approximates very closely that of an adult. Also by age five the child is able to comprehend most syntactic structures. The more difficult grammatical structures, i.e., jokes, double meaning words, and sarcasm continue to gradually develop until mastered at approximately 10 years of age.

Researchers such as Wolfram and Christian (1975) state that non-standard dialect is rule governed and therefore a valid mode of communication. Teachers continue to judge such dialect utterances as if they are substandard. Thus educational placement may be determined by teachers whose perceptions of the child's oral language may be inappropriate.

Listener Perception and Dialect

In a recent study of listener attitudes of general American speech, New England dialect, and Appalachian dialect, Rudd and Mulac

(1977) found that Appalachian dialect rated the lowest in socio-intellectual status. Gonzalez (1974) believes that when a child's linguistic system is rejected, the school is essentially rejecting the linguistic and cultural heritage under which the child learns to speak. This rejection causes alienation of the dialect speaking child from the school system. The child literally questions the credibility of the educational system.

Labov (1967) points out that one cause of teacher rejection of dialect is based on the premise that many of these teachers grew up in culturally diverse communities and succeeded academically by learning standard English. This makes these particular teachers more intolerant of non-standard usage than most middle-class standard English speakers.

This discussion does not intimate that the culturally different and poor child should not learn standard English. The child must learn to communicate in the mainstream communication modality if he is to be competitive with the middle class educationally, vocationally, and socially. It must be stressed that the manner in which the educational system chooses to deal with the culturally different and poor child's communication has serious implications on the development of a healthy self concept and a desire to achieve in the existing educational establishment.

School Phobia

Often it has been said that societal efforts for the culturally different and poor have been wasted because of a seeming lack of interest, poor school attendance, and a high school dropout rate resulting in adult welfare recipients.

Looff (1971) completed research with children in Appalachia. His study indicates that many culturally different and poor youth develop many emotionally deviant behaviors when entering the middle-class school for the first time. He stressed that many of these children became non-verbal when they realized their communication system was different from what was expected. Accompanying elective mutism was minor illness and chronic absences. Looff used the term school phobia to incorporate all of these symptoms. His research concluded that children exhibiting school phobia symptoms eventually became school dropouts.

The school system or teacher may possess the following set of expectations that contribute to the dropout rate of the culturally different and poor student. Teachers may expect the dialect speaker to function according to middle-class standards while never experiencing standard English. Teacher expectations are as follows:

1. Comprehension of spoken standard English
2. Comprehension of written standard English
3. Expression, both oral and written, in standard English

While the child's language is sufficient to handle his needs within the dialect community, it is different from the standard English of the school system. As a result, the child must translate the spoken language of the teacher and make his own language match that of the teacher's standard English. Anastasiow (1976) in agreement with Labov stresses that the major fallacy is the school's assumption that the child will come to school understanding the spoken English of the teacher and further that the teacher is not responsible for teaching the child the standard English communication system of the school.

Obviously one of the contributing factors of school failure among the culturally different and poor population is the lack of attainment of academic skills. Previous chapters in this book have discussed treatment methods such as eradication and laissez-faire. These methods either devaluate the individual's culture and communication system or ignore it. Certainly these treatment methods are not effective in creating positive education advancement for this population under consideration.

Employability

As previously stated, listener perceptions of dialect speakers form a limiting assumption about the dialect speaker's intellectual abilities. This assumption is most inhibiting to job attainment commensurate with the skills possessed by the individual. Therefore, the dialect speaker must settle for a lower paying or less prestigious employment. Adler (1981) states the employability problem in this manner:

> In general it may be said that many economically poor speakers retain the linguistic and paralinguistic patterns of their culture; i.e., poor Blacks continue to use Black English dialect and poor Appalachians continue to use mountain English dialect. And, as suggested, such dialectal usage often penalizes the user in the middle-class "market place" where standard English is assumed to be the only proper English dialect.

Bidialectalism

An alternative to the eradication and laissez-faire method is bidialectalism. This approach makes no effort to eradicate the student's non-standard dialect. Unlike the laissez-faire approach, bidialectalism teaches standard usage via contrastive analysis. Dialect is given equal status with standard English to equip the student with control over two dialect systems that function within his communcation environment. It also acquaints the student with a value system to determine which dialect is appropriate for varying communication settings.

Proponents of bidialectalism or the difference theorists believe that upon school entrance all children possess an extensive linguistic facility, a large vocabulary, and an efficient means of oral communication. The research of the difference theorists clearly supports the fact that culturally different children are not handicapped in the area of linguistics unless the handicap is measured in terms of their control of standard English.

Brandes and Brewer (1977) note that children speaking dialects of English have a very effective method of communication with their peers and family. They have a rich vocabulary, an extensive syntax, and a consistent phonological pattern as well as an established paralinguistic system.

Bidialectalism and Research

Research to support or contradict the bidialectal method is sparse. Leaverton (1969) in Chicago used pattern drills to formulate a reading program for black first graders. In this program dialect readers were utilized to contrast and compare the differences between "everyday" and "school" talk.

Rystrom (1970) did research with black first graders in Georgia and California. Children received bidialect training in oral language while at the same time receiving formal reading instruction. No significant differences were noted between the experimental group or control group. Rystrom believed that the concurrent oral language and reading instruction may have been confusing for the children. These findings substantiate the belief that bidialectal instruction should take place before initiation of formalized reading instruction. The reader must be aware that oral language is a primary linguistic skill that is a prerequisite to the secondary linguistic skills of reading and writing.

The Clayton (1974) study of kindergarten through third grade children in Morgan County, Tennessee, was the first successful program used with the rural Appalachian population. Two important findings in the Clayton study were observed. First, dialect speaking children became more verbal in the reguar classroom. Second, with the increase of verbal expression, teacher opinions in relation to the children's learning aptitude changed in a more positive fashion.

A two-year program with Head Start (Adler, 1979) in Knox County, Tennessee, utilizing bidialectal language teaching strategies as compared to unidialectal language instruction was implemented. Findings indicated that standard English is more effectively learned by culturally different and poor children when they are taught by the bidialectal-bicultural teaching strategy than by conventional language arts methods. It must be noted that a rigorous program of inservice training for regular classroom teachers and parent education is paramount for the acceptance and implementation of the bidialectal teaching method.

TRADITIONAL ROLES OF THE SPEECH-LANGUAGE PATHOLOGIST

The School Setting — Historical Perspective

During the 1950's through the early 1970's the speech-language pathologist's role was one of screening, diagnostic testing, and treatment of speech, hearing, and language disorders. These disorders were mainly related to faulty or incomplete learning, brain damage, emotional problems or mental retardation. This model provided a framework for viewing speech and language problems as deficient due to organic or functional etiology and led to a treatment model of therapeutic remediation and correction. Speech-language pathologists in the public school setting usually worked independently from the rest of the educational staff, taking children out of the classroom for thirty- or sixty-minute sessions once or twice a week. Therapy goals and student progress was shared informally with the classroom teacher with a formal report possibly included in the student's record. Parents received a progress report or had an occasional conference with the pathologist periodically during the school year.

Dialect speaking children were labeled deficient in the areas of speech and language according to data obtained from standardized testing designed for the middle-class population. Dialect children were placed in therapy to eradicate the dialect replacing it with standard English.

Early in her professional career, this author operated under this framework. Children who were black or Appalachian dialect speakers were diagnosed as having deficits via standardized tests normed for the white middle-class standard English speaker. Dialect speaking children received therapy to eradicate their dialect. These children were taught that what they said (vocabulary) and how they said it (morphology, syntax, and phonology) was wrong. Standard English, they were told, was the only acceptable mode of communication. Carryover of standard English outside the therapy setting was rarely accomplished. Most children would perform pattern drills in standard English such as those found in the Distar Language Program; however, non-standard dialect was almost always used in the classroom and at home. Later these children were dismissed for lack of progress. Little was accomplished other than a small increase of vocabulary skills. Frustration on the part of the pathologist was evidenced and the children obviously felt a sense of failure. A colleague chose to operate under the laissez-faire method. The need to learn standard English was realized; however, the teaching effort was deemed impossible due to the strong influence of the dialect and culture within the community. All of the children were treated unfairly. Most had academic problems in part because of the lack of facility with standard English. Our treatment methods, either eradication or laissez-faire, were not appropriate for this population.

Current Litigation

Two important pieces of litigation have affected how the speech-language pathologist functions within the public school setting. Garrard (1978) states that the Education of All Handicapped Children Act, Public Law 94-142, passed in 1975, was a legislative landmark that had the greatest impact in the area of special education of which our profession is a part.

Under PL 94-142, all children must receive culturally non-biased assessment. Children must be evaluated in terms of their culture and dialect. No longer can a dialect be labeled a deficiency. As speech-langauge pathologists, we must provide appropriate assessment measures and appropriate treatment methods. A dialect speaking child can no longer be considered handicapped based on tests normed solely for the white middleclass child.

This certainly does not mean that this population can be ignored by members of our profession. The role of the speech-language pathologist is one of a facilitator of communication skills for all children, not only the ones formally on our caseload labeled as possessing communication deficiencies, but also those children manifesting communication differences. When a child completes his public school education, he is expected to possess competencies in academic subjects and oral communication skills. These skills enable the student to obtain gainful employment or to pursue vocational or college education. The main goal of public education is to train individuals to be effective, contributing members of society. If the educational system cannot accomplish this goal for the culturally different and poor child, then educators need to reevaluate their techniques and make mandatory changes within the system.

Another important piece of litigation having impact for dialect speakers was the Ann Arbor Decision. Parents of black school children in Ann Arbor, Michigan, brought suit against the school system because their children were not learning to read. Federal Judge Charles Joiner (Bountress, 1980) stated that one of the most urgent problems to be addressed for children speaking social dialects was the lack of sensitivity of the teachers to the dialect. He further stated that teachers have inadequately taught these children to speak standard English. The Ann Arbor Decision ordered the educators to teach standard English. Educators must be aware of reading and dialect mismatch in educating black dialect speaking children. This decision implies consideration be given all dialect speaking children in all educational settings.

It is the function of the speech-language pathologist to help develop, along with the classroom teacher, an effective bidialectal and bicultural teaching program.

Speech-Language Pathologist — Personal Evaluation

The speech-language pathologist, whether in the school or clinic setting, must honestly evaluate his own feelings and biases before working with the culturally different and poor child. The following self-evaluative questions were developed by the California Department of Special Education (1971). During a conference concerning appropriate programs for the culturally diverse, the committee stated that speech-language pathologists and other special educators attempting to educate minority children must realize that they can be part of the caste system which perpetuates the low status of culturally different and poor children. If there are positive responses to the following questions with exception of No. 8, then the speech-language pathologist should not work with these children. Another colleague should undertake the task of working with this population. Although the committee's focus was the Spanish population of California, it is believed that the questions are applicable to any dialect or cultural diversity.

1. To what extent do you permit the pigmentation of skin or neighborhood address or Spanish surname of the minority child to influence the assessment of the adequacy of a child's speech and language pattern?
2. How often does your diagnosis of cultural deprivation assume a correlation among factors of skin color, IQ level, phonemic system, and linguistic behavior?
3. Is your approach possibly condescending so that the minority child recognizes your rejection and discomfort and in turn feels humiliation, unworthiness, and hostility?
4. Is your approach dishonest from the very onset because you do not expect the child with a cultural difference to put forth great effort or initiative to perform well or even achieve average success?
5. Do you unconsciously apply double standards that excuse poor work because the child is poor and black?
6. Are you aware of the circular reasoning that restricts the behavior of the child tagged as culturally deficient and traps the therapist in a cycle of over-simplifying lessons with preconceived low objectives to meet predetermined needs and deficits?
7. Do your beliefs concerning middle-class standards of speech inhibit full appreciation and respect for the minority child's linguistic system that ultimately denegates the minority child's social dialect?

8. Or is your attitude one of genuine concern and interest, not because the minority child is poor or dark skinned or speaks non-standard English, but because he is respected as a human being?

Professional Skills of the Speech-Language Pathologist

Before a speech-language pathologist can begin to work with the culturally diverse, he must possess certain competencies. The American Speech and Hearing Association's Code of Ethics states that the member must not provide services for which he or she has not been properly trained, i.e., not had the necessary course work and supervised practicum. Therefore, when a pathologist offers professional services to any individual, he should possess all relevant information concerning the client including knowledge relevant to the client's culture and dialect.

The speech-language pathologist must be able to diagnose speech and language that is different from speech that is deviant. In order to do this the pathologist must have a thorough knowledge of the phonology, syntax, and lexicon of the dialect. A knowledge of applicable standardized tests must also be possessed by the pathologist. Items to consider when using such diagnostic tools include how the particular test was standardized, what was the normative population, is dialect taken into consideration in the scoring procedure, will this test give an accurate profile of the individual's strengths and weaknesses, or can this test be used for item analysis only?

Testing

An informal question and answer session may only serve to silence the child, making it difficult to gather enough spontaneous speech to analyze. In light of this, many speech-language pathologists resort solely to the use of standardized tests which present another set of problems. Musselwhite (1983) believes that some tests are culturally biased because they present pictures and vocabulary familiar to the middle-class child but outside the range of a lower-class child's experience. It is important to understand that a test is automatically biased just because lower-class children make lower scores on it than their middle-class peers. Much depends on what the test is supposed to measure. If testing indicates that minority-group children consistently score lower than middle-class children, then the pathologist needs to question whether the test is measuring language ability or middle-class word knowledge.

Another difficulty in administering tests involves the influence of extraneous variables on a child's performance. If we do get the child's best performance, the score should be disregarded. These children may be afraid to interact with strangers. They may not be motivated to perform well. They also may not understand the test directions and are afraid to ask questions. These points are very important to consider when testing any child, especially a culturally different and poor child. The speech-language pathologist must give the child the opportunity to acclimate himself to the setting, the test, and the tester.

The development of local norms is suggested by Evard and Sabers (1979) to increase validity of tests for the culturally different population. Comparison of both standard norms and community norms is advocated. Those children having language disorders relative to their peer group could be identified by use of local norms with this group requiring direct therapeutic intervention. The implication here is that these children do not learn those behaviors to which they were presumably exposed. The standardized norms help identify those children with language differences whose needs could not be met by more general programs such as the bidialectal method of teaching standard English in the regular classroom setting.

The state of Tennessee has an implementation manual to be used for student screening and assessment of all handicapping conditions applicable to Public Law 94-142. This author assumes that other states have like documents for implementation in order that handicapped children are accurately screened, diagnosed, and placed in appropriate programs. Such manuals contain information as to what constitutes a diagnostic evaluation for speech and language assessment. The following is a model used by this author working primarily with the Appalachian population. Some of the tests utilized were not the best but what was available under budget constraints. The speech-language pathologist must realize that the ideal diagnostic battery may not always be available and must be flexible and innovative with the use of existing tools.

For speech screening, the Photo Articulation Test was used (Interstate Print and Publishers). This is a photo identification task that probes both the vowels and consonants in IMF positions of words. It also contains a sequence picture story to elicit a conversation sample. The photographs are easier for the young child to identify versus a two-dimension line drawing of pictures. This test was normed locally for Appalachian dialect and black dialect. The test was scored with consideration of dialect. Another speech screening measure used is the Fluharty Preschool Language Screening Test used with the kindergarten or 4-year olds. The speech section probes initial and final consonants. The scoring manual has norms for black dialect speakers. Appalachian norms again had to be established.

For speech diagnostics, an oral facial exam, a hearing screening, an articulation test, and a conversation sample is required. Again local norms for the Templin Darley Test of Articulation were established. The articulation test was scored with comparison of standardized norms and peer or local norms. The same procedure was used for the conversation sample. The author found it easier to make a phonetic transcription of a taped sample rather than to take the sample in writing during the diagnostic session allowing for several listenings of the tape when necessary.

Language diagnostics include measures of receptive vocabulary, syntax, and morphology. Expressive measures consist of mean length of utterance, syntax, semantics, pragmatics, and morphology. Finally, measures of auditory perception including selective attention, discrimination, memory, sequencing, association, and integration complete the linguistic diagnostic profile. This author has used the Peabody Picture Vocabulary Test Revised for measuring receptive vocabulary. The Illinois Test of Psycholinguistic Abilities is used; however, local norms for Appalachian dialect were established for the Grammatic Closure Subtest. The Test of Language Development covers areas of receptive and expressive vocabulary, sentence imitation, syntax, morphology, auditory discrimination, and word articulation. In the administration manual of the test, there is a section on establishing local norms to obtain a culture fair assessment. The Daily Language Facility Test probes vocabulary, pronunciation, and grammar. Here the child is shown three pictures at a time and asked to tell a story about them. This measure can be used alone or in combination with other tests. It gives a speech sample that can be analyzed and compared with morphology and syntax in other formal measures. A spontaneous speech sample is also necessary. This author has found that peer conversations at play, in the lunchroom, or in the classroom give good indication of morphological and syntactical structures readily used by the child.

It is the pathologist's responsibility to be thoroughly familiar with ancillary services available within the local community when attempting to meet the needs of the culturally different and poor population. These agencies could include the public health department, department of human services, community action agencies, and the like. The pathologist needs to know referral procedures for each agency as much time is wasted waiting for appropriate service when incorrect referral procedures are used. Often the child has medical, psychological, or other problems that have direct influence on hearing, speech, and language problems. It is within the domain of the speech-language pathologist to ensure that the child receives appropriate care.

Pupil Placement

As mandated by PL 94-142, the speech-language pathologist is a part of a multidisciplinary team. He/she is required within the public school setting to assess the communication needs of handicapped children. He/she must ensure that the education of the child is appropriate. It is reasonable to expect that observations and testing results of a child's language skills should concur, for example, with verbal measures used by the school psychologist. If not, then there is a problem either with the pathologist's assessment or the psychological assessment for that particular child.

This author was part of a multidisciplinary team to consider resource room placement for a black first grader. The classroom teacher made the diagnostic referral on the basis of unintelligibility of the child's oral language and low vocabulary skills. On all measures of communication assessment the child performed appropriately for his age level. Articulation testing revealed appropriate black dialect phonology. The child was the only black student in this particular first grade classroom. The teacher believed that this child should speak standard English as did the rest of the children in the class. The school psychologist stated that the child possessed normal performance abilities as evidenced by psychometric testing; however, there was a large discrepancy in the verbal scale performance of the testing. The pathologist questioned the validity of the verbal portion of the test. Upon request, the psychologist listened to an informal conversation with the student in question about his football hero, Mean Joe Green. What the psychologist heard was a very verbal child with dialect appropriate utterances. The psychological report was changed to reflect the child's facility of black dialect. During the M-team meeting, the child was placed in another first grade class where there were several other black children. The new teacher was more sensitive to dialect and could teach standard English in a nonderogatory manner. Resource room placement was considered inappropriate.

Another example of similar nature involved a student who attended a small rural kindergarten class and transferred to an urban school at the beginning of first grade. During speech screening he recognized one of the speech pathologists. He said excitedly, "Teacher ain't y'all proud to be a seein me in this here fine school?" To ease the move to a new school the parents told the boy his new school was bigger and had better facilities. The rural school population was made up of low-income Appalachian dialect speaking children. In fact, many of the faculty members came from similar backgrounds and were sensitive to the dialect. This was not the case in the urban school. His peers and teachers made fun of his speech. This "fine new school" became a threatening place. The child developed school phobia. Due to chronic absences he became a referral to the resource teacher. Although he passed the speech and language screening, a language diagnostic was also obtained. Using local norms, the language skills were appropriate for his age and level of functioning. Both psychological and resource testing indicated average intelligence and skills. Resource room placement was not appropriate. The classroom teacher was counseled regarding dialect. This teacher permitted the pathologist to include bidialectal teaching with the regular weekly speech improvement lessons. The psychologist used the boy's knowledge of farm life on a class field trip. His classmates were awed with the boy's knowledge of animal care, milking, planting, and baling hay. These intervention methods helped in making the child feel accepted. He finished the year with above-average grades and, with a small amount of bidialectalism, acquired the ability to code switch from dialect to standard English.

The speech-language pathologist must prevent inappropriate placement. No matter how hard we try to disguise it, the resource room still has the connotation of the place for those who cannot succeed in the regular classroom, i.e., the slow learner. Whether the child spends a few months or several years in the resource room, this information is noted on the student's permanent records. This can be very stigmatizing for the child.

Treatment

There will be dialect speaking children in the public school setting that will have deficiencies that require therapeutic management. Take, for example, the black child who omits the [s] phoneme in all positions of words. The speech-language pathologist must be aware that when the child reaches phrase, sentence, and carryover level the final [s] is omitted in black dialect in words that connote quantity. When judging therapy progress, the pathologist must consider dialect usage. Other children within the same therapy group who are standard English speakers may become confused with the acceptance of dialect utterances for the black child, yet not from the standard English speakers. How can the pathologist manage this situation? The only satisfactory solution for this author is the initiation of the bidialectic approach in the therapy setting. The students are made aware of the culture and dialect differences via comparing and contrasting dialect with standard English. The students are satisfied with this explanation, learn about other cultures and dialects within their community, and compare and contrast home and school talk. In this manner the dialect speaker is able to learn standard English, and learn when it is appropriate to use dialect and standard English. Once the pathologist is satisfied that the dialect speaker has mastered the [s] phoneme through conversation level, the student can be dismissed as corrected. Standard English is then taught in the classroom via the bidialectal method by the regular classroom teacher.

Another example of the use of the bidialectal method in the therapy setting was seen with a group of moderate-to-severe articulation disordered Appalachian dialect speaking children. Upon initiation of therapy, this author operated under the eradication philosophy. During the first year the articulation improved yet the dialect remained. During that year one child remarked that his father and grandfather talked that way and they were not wrong. The next year the bidialectal method was instituted in therapy. This method did not cause the children to question the intelligence or propriety of their parent's communication system or have a power struggle with the speech-language pathologist. At the end of the school year the children had corrected all articulation errors and were able to use both standard English and Appalachian dialect when appropriate. In this author's opinion, the use of the bidialectal approach is the only method that can handle such situations in the therapy setting.

UNCONVENTIONAL ROLES OF THE SPEECH-LANGUAGE PATHOLOGIST

Consultants to Classroom Teachers

If culturally different and poor children do not warrant direct service from the speech-language pathologist in the therapy setting, the pathologist cannot ignore the communication needs of this population. As stated in the initial portion of this chapter, oral language is the basis for academic skill acquisition. Unfortunately, for most dialect speakers upon school entrance there is a mismatch between the valid linguistic system possessed by the child and the standard English used by the teacher and found within the curricula. This is most evident when the child begins formal reading instruction. Hargis (1982) states four principles that must be considered for effective reading instruction. This author believes these principles are vital and deserve serious consideration when dealing with dialect speaking students. They are as follows:

1. The communication with which children are familiar should be reflected in the composition of language they are learning to read.
2. Reading material used must be within experience and linguistic thresholds that each child brings to the instructional setting.
3. One cannot comprehend through listening, language that relates unfamiliar experience and one cannot read unfamiliar language.
4. Only language conversationally familiar should be used for instruction in beginning reading.

Without consideration of Hargis's four principles, the dialect speaking child is forced into a no-win situation. Without learning the language of the textbooks, the child becomes a curriculum casualty.

How then can the speech-language pathologist serve these children? In a recent attitude survey to assess the strengths and weaknesses of the ongoing speech-language program in a rural county of Tennessee, classroom teachers were asked if children should learn standard English. Ninety-seven percent of the teachers strongly agreed that the students need facility in standard English usage. Through teacher training sessions, the speech-language pathologist can institute the bidialectic teaching method used by the regular classroom teacher. The techniques must be made simple to execute and also fit into the existing curriculum. The pathologist can arrange to do demonstration teaching initially on a weekly basis with teacher followup throughout the remainder of the week. When the classroom teacher feels competent within the structure of the teaching method, then the pathologist can meet weekly with the teacher to discuss any problems and future lessons. Again, the key to the success of this method is the ability to incorporate the bidialectal method and teaching techniques into the existing curricula. Demonstration teaching by the speech-language pathologist has a hidden benefit. With their large caseload, pathologists rarely have the opportunity to observe their students in the classroom setting. Here the pathologist can determine whether or not communication strategies are being used by the child outside the therapy setting.

Bidialectal Teaching Strategies

The teaching method of bidialectalism is based on the principles of contrastive analysis. Adler (1979) states that learning the different features of both dialect and standard English should begin with ear training.

In a contrastive auditory program, the contrast between the standard and non-standard English form is presented, and the auditor is asked to repeat the standard form. In this way the phonological syntactic and lexical differences between standard and non-standard dialects can be distinguished.

There are five steps in contrastive analysis. The first phase is presentation. The teacher presents both the non-standard and standard versions and compares and contrasts them for the students. For example, the teacher would say: "He run fast" and "He runs fast." Next, discrimination drills should be used for the students to hear differences between the two forms.

Example: Teacher -   He run fast.   Student - different
                     He runs fast.
                     He run fast.   Student - same
                     He run fast.

Identification drills are utilized next for the student to delineate the dialect response from the standard English response.

Example: Teacher -   He runs fast.   Student - standard
                     He run fast.   Student - non-standard

Often the student can correctly identify utterances of dialect and standard English; then he is required to orally translate a standard utterance into nonstandard or vice-versa. These are called translation drills.

After the student has acquired mastery in translation drills, response drills are employed. Here, if the teacher makes a nonstandard utterance, the student is expected to respond with a non-standard reply. The same procedure would be expected for an utterance in standard English.

Example: Teacher -   He run fast.   Student - No, he don't.
                     He runs fast. Student - No, he doesn't.

Through contrastive analysis procedure, the primary goal is teaching standard English speaking and writing skills to culturally different children. To reiterate, utilization of this approach bases itself on the linguistic system the child brings to the classroom. Change is made via contrastive analysis in order that the child can function competitively with his peers in a manner that in no way negates the value of the culturally different and poor child's language culture.

Parents and the Speech-Language Pathologist

Speech-language pathologists must operate on the belief that all parents are concerned about their child's progress. Low-income parents may lack the time or knowledge to express this concern. Coming to school or a clinic setting may be a threatening situation for the parent. In this case, the pathologist must be able to communicate to the parent that he possesses skills that are valid and necessary in training his child.

Home visits offer a wealth of information about the child for the pathologist. It is within the home environment where we can demonstrate to the parent how to structure language habilitation procedures in a naturalistic environment. A daily household routine, for example setting the table, can serve as a means to teach sorting, counting, matching, and oral language to the child. It is in the home environment where the pathologist can train the parent to model appropriate responses, expand the child's utterances, and create effective learning via daily routines.

Parent weekly support groups where parents can freely discuss their relationship with their children, attitudes concerning disciplines, etc., offer another means of effective parent education for the speech-language pathologist. As parents learn from each other, they are better equipped to understand and cope with upgrading the child's communication skills. Webster (1966) says that parent meetings such as mentioned above provide parents with three vital aids:

1. Important information about the child's specific disorder
2. Opportunities for parents to experiment with tools for promoting better communication
   a. trying to understand the child's feelings and verbalizing this understanding
   b. trying to accept the child's feeling, even when the behavior is unacceptable
   c. allowing the child time with his parents when they can concentrate on communicating
   d. giving the child a chance to communicate at times when he feels success and satisfaction
   e. attempting to communicate with the child on his own level
3. A chance to verbalize frankly about vital issues in their relationships and forces that motivate them

The speech-language pathologist should incorporate the school psychologist, special educator, and social worker and teacher in the parent groups when appropriate. All disciplines have much expertise to contribute in creating a successful positive learning environment for the child.

Parents should also become active participants within the therapy setting, instead of silent observers. As an active participant, the parent would become an aid to the pathologist. This author has utilized parents in this manner for several years with excellent success. In this situation, the parent has the opportunity to learn various behavior management techniques as well as pragmatic language habilitation methods. These parents were able to observe the functioning level of their child with respect to the other children in the group. Through this experience the parents were able to establish reasonable goals and expectations for their children.

Clinic Setting — The Private Practitioner

In general the private practitioner does not serve the neglected population. The pathologist is a business person and cannot afford to serve those who cannot pay for services. The pathologist, however, may serve the culturally different and poor in contract programs with ancillary agencies within the local community. When this is the situation, the pathologist must take measures similar to his public school counterpart to ensure that the client receives a culturally fair evaluation. The client must be made to feel at ease in the diagnostic setting. If the client is a child, involve the parent in the diagnostic process to help elicit conversation samples and judge performance levels on testing measures. Observe the parent-child interaction. If possible, the pathologist should evaluate the child in familiar surroundings such as home, day care facility, or nursery school. Always ask the parent if information obtained during assessment is typical of the child's ability.

The pathologist should act as a consultant with these ancillary agencies to train staff members in language habilitation strategies. Cultural and dialect differences should be stressed with implementation of bidialectal teaching methods in order that the young child can learn standard English.

Clinic Setting — University Training Facility

The university clinic has the unique responsibility of training future speech-language pathologists and meeting client needs in the areas of diagnostic evaluation and treatment. In order to obtain competency in working with culturally diverse populations, the university curricula must include appropriate course work and supervised practica as prescribed by the American Speech and Hearing Association's Code of Ethics. Course work should include basic language development, social and cultural aspects that influence language development and language learning, standard and nonstandard forms of English, diagnostic instruments for culturally fair evaluation, and teaching methods for standard English.

Ideas and methods taught in the classroom must carry over to the clinic practica. Students need experience in testing and report writing reflecting awareness of dialect. Outreach programs should be established in day care and nursery schools to facilitate acquisition of standard English utilizing bidialectal methods. Often local, state or federal grants are available to help fund such efforts. Ongoing research is always necessary in dealing with new methods for teaching the culturally diverse populations.

CONCLUSION

The role of the speech-language pathologist working with the culturally different and poor population must be that of a communication facilitator. Both in the clinic setting and in the public schools the pathologist must ensure that the individual receives an appropriate assessment and treatment method in view of the culture and dialect.

This author advocates the use of bidialectal philosophy and teaching strategies to facilitate the appropriate use of standard English. In order to implement bidialectal methods, the pathologist must be an effective trainer of teachers who works daily with the culturally different and poor population. To accomplish this goal, the pathologist must expand his/her influence from the therapy room to the classroom, community, and home environment of the dialect speaker. Our profession is one part of the total educational process which equips the culturally different and poor population to become self sufficient and contributing members of society.

REFERENCES

Adler, S. *Poverty Children and Their Language*. New York: Grune & Stratton, 1979.

Adler, S. "Social Dialect and Literacy: The Relationship Among Talking, Reading, and Writing in Culturally Different and Poor Children." See Part I.

Anastasiow, N., and Hanes, M. *Language Patterns of Poverty Children*. Springfield: Charles C Thomas, 1976.

Bountress, N. G. The Ann Arbor Decision: Implications for Speech-Language Pathologists. *ASHA*, 22, 543-544, 1980.

Brandes, P. H., and Brewer, J. *Dialect Clash in America: Issues and Answers.* Metuchen, N. J.: The Scarecrow Press, 1977.

California Department of Special Education. Special Language Programming for Exceptional Children with Language Disorders. ERIC Document ED 051618, 1971.

Clayton, Kenneth. "Evaluation of the Effectiveness of Short Term Utilization of a Budgeted Method of Teaching Language to White Appalachian Elementary School Children." Unpublished Master's Thesis, University of Tennessee, 1974.

Evard, B. L., and Sabers, D. L. Speech and Language Testing with Distinct Ethnic-Racial Groups: A Survey of Procedures for Improving Validity. *Journal of Speech and Hearing Disorders*, 44, 271-281, 1979.

Garrard, K. R. The Changing Role of the Speech and Hearing Professionals in Public Education. *ASHA*, 91, February, 1978.

Gonzalez, R. In Hess, K. ERIC Document ED 098602, 1974.

Hargis, C. H. *Teaching Reading to Handicapped Children.* Denver: Love, 16, 1982.

Labov, W. Some Sources of Reading Problems for Negro Speakers of Nonstandard English. In A. Frazier (Ed.). *New Directions in Elementary English.* Champaign, Ill.: National Council of Teachers of English, 1967.

Leaverton, L. Dialectal Readers; Rational and Value. Paper presented at Preconvention Institute of the International Reading Association. Atlantic City, N.J., 1971.

Looff, D. H. *Appalachia's Children.* Lexington, Ky.: The University Press of Kentucky, 1971.

Mulac, A., and Rudd, M. J. Effects of Selected Regional American Dialects upon Regional Audience Members. *Communication Monographs*, 44, 185-195, 1977.

Musselwhite, C. R. Pluralistic Assessment in Speech-Language Pathology: Use of Oral Norms in the Placement Process. Language, Speech, and Hearing Service in Schools, 14, 29-37, 1983.

Rystrom, R. C. Dialect Training and Reading: A Further Look. *Reading Research Quarterly*, 40, 581-599, 1970.

Venezky, R. L., Non-standard Language and Reading. *Elementary English*, 47, 334-345, 1970.

Webster, E. J. Parent Counseling by Speech Pathologists and Audiologists. *Journal of Speech and Hearing Disorders*, 31, 331-340, 1966.

Wolfram, W., and Christian, D. *Sociolinguistic Variables in Appalachian Dialects.* Arlington, Va.: Center for Applied Linguistics, 1975.

APPENDIX CONTENTS

Appendix IA

DIAGNOSTIC DATA

A. PUBLIC SCHOOL SAMPLES

THE first two articulation score sheets include an example of black dialect and Appalachian dialect respectively. Without consideration of dialect, these two profiles would be labeled deficient, requiring therapeutic management by the speech-language pathologist according to standardized norms of phonological acquisition.

The third articulation score sheet is another typical example of Appalachian dialect that does require therapy intervention by the pathologist.

In all three cases acquisition of standard English is a valid skill needed to be mastered by the student.

PAT RECORDING SHEET

		Year	Month	Day
Name	James Parker	Date	83	9	15
School	Midtown Elementary	Birth	76	6	2
Grade	2	Age	7	3	

Key: Omission (–); substitution (write phonetic symbol of sound substituted); severity of distortion (D1), (D2), (D3); ability to imitate (circle symbol or error).

Black English

Sound	Photograph	1	2	3	Vowels, Diph.			Comments
	I				**III**			
s	saw, pencil, house	x	x	x	aʊ	house	x	f /θ, b/v, w/hw –
s bl	spoon, skates, stars	x	x	x				dialect appropriate
z	zipper, scissors, keys	x	x	–				
ʃ	shoe, station, fish	x	x	x	u	shoe	x	
tʃ	chair, matches, sandwich	x	x	x				
dʒ	jars, angels, orange	x	x	x				
t	table, potatoes, hat	x	x	x	æ	hat	x	
d	dog, ladder, bed	x	x	x	ɔ	dog	x	
n	nails, bananas, can	x	x	x	ə	bananas	x	
l	lamp, balloons, bell	x	x	x	ɛ	bell	x	
l bl	blocks, clock, flag	x	x	x	ɑ	blocks	x	
θ	thumb, toothbrush, teeth	f	f	f	i	teeth	x	
r	radio, carrots, car	x	x	–				
r bl	brush, crayons, train	x	x	x	e	train	x	
k	cat, crackers, cake	x	x	x	ɚ-ə	crackers	x	
g	gun, wagon, egg	x	x	x	ʌ	gun	x	
	II							
f	fork, elephant, knife	x	x	x				
v	vacuum, TV, stove	b	b	b	ju	vacuum	x	
p	pipe, apples, cup	x	x	x	aɪ	pipe	x	
b	book, baby, bathtub	x	x	x	ʊ	book	x	
m	monkey, hammer, comb	x	x	x	o	comb	x	**SCORE**
w-hw	witch, flowers, whistle	x	x	w	ɪ	witch	x	
	I							*Sounds*
ð	this, that, feathers, bathe	d	v	v				I Tongue _____
h-ŋ	hanger, hanger, swing	x	x	x				II Lip _____
j	yes, thank you	x	x					III Vowels _____
ʒ	measure, beige	x	x		ɔɪ	boy	x	Total _____
	(story)				ɚ-ɜ	bird	x	

PAT RECORDING SHEET

		Year	Month	Day
Name	Mary Jane Little	Date	83	9	15
School	Midtown	Birth	75	8	20
Grade	3	Age	8	0	

Key: Omission (–); substitution (write phonetic symbol of sound substituted); severity of distortion (D1), (D2), (D3); ability to imitate (circle symbol or error).

Appalachian Dialect

Sound	Photograph	1	2	3	Vowels, Diph.		Comments
	I				**III**		
s	saw, pencil, house	x	x	x	aʊ house	x	No errors – dialect
s bl	spoon, skates, stars	x	x	x			appropriate
z	zipper, scissors, keys	x	x	x			
ʃ	shoe, station, fish	x	x	x	u shoe	x	
tʃ	chair, matches, sandwich	x	x	x			
dʒ	jars, angels, orange	x	x	x			
t	table, potatoes, hat	x	x	x	æ hat	x	
d	dog, ladder, bed	x	x	x	ɔ dog	x	
n	nails, bananas, can	x	x	x	ə bananas	x	
l	lamp, balloons, bell	x	x	x	ɛ bell	x	
l bl	blocks, clock, flag	x	x	x	ɑ blocks	x	
θ	thumb, toothbrush, teeth	f	f	f	i teeth	x	
r	radio, carrots, car	x	x	x			
r bl	brush, crayons, train	x	x	x	e train	x	
k	cat, crackers, cake	x	x	x	ɚ–ə crackers	x	
g	gun, wagon, egg	x	x	x	ʌ gun	x	
	II						
f	fork, elephant, knife	x	x	x			
v	vacuum, TV, stove	b	b	b	ju vacuum	x	
p	pipe, apples, cup	x	x	x	aɪ pipe	x	
b	book, baby, bathtub	x	x	x	ʊ book	x	
m	monkey, hammer, comb	x	x	x	o comb	x	
w-hw	witch, flowers, whistle	x	x	w	ɪ witch	x	SCORE
	I						
ð	this, that, feathers, bathe	d	v	v			Sounds
h-ŋ	hanger, hanger, swing	x	g	g			I Tongue_____
j	yes, thank you	x	x				II Lip _____
ʒ	measure, beige	x	dʒ		ɔɪ boy	x	III Vowels_____
	(story)				ɚ–ə bird	x	Total _____

PAT RECORDING SHEET

	Year	Month	Day
Name **Bobbie Sue Stevens** Date	83	9	15
School **Midtown** Birth	75	7	1
Grade **3** Age	8	2	

Key: Omission (–); substitution (write phonetic symbol of sound substituted); severity of distortion (D1), (D2), (D3); ability to imitate (circle symbol or error).

Appalachian Dialect

Sound	Photograph	1	2	3	Vowels, Diph.		Comments
	I				**III**		
s	saw, pencil, house	x	x	–	aʊ house		f/θ, b/v, d/ð, v/ð –
s bl	spoon, skates, stars	x	x	x			dialect appropriate
z	zipper, scissors, keys	x	x	–			
ʃ	shoe, station, fish	x	x	x	u shoe		
tʃ	chair, matches, sandwich	x	x	x			
dʒ	jars, angels, orange	x	x	x			
t	table, potatoes, hat	x	x	x	æ hat		
d	dog, ladder, bed	x	x	x	ɔ dog		
n	nails, bananas, can	x	x	x	ə bananas		
l	lamp, balloons, bell	x	x	–	ɛ bell		
l bl	blocks, clock, flag	w	w	w	ɑ blocks		
θ	thumb, toothbrush, teeth	f	f	f	i teeth		
r	radio, carrots, car	w	w	–			
r bl	brush, crayons, train	w	w	w	e train		
k	cat, crackers, cake	x	x	x	ɚ-ɔ crackers		
g	gun, wagon, egg	x	x	x	ʌ gun		
	II						
f	fork, elephant, knife	x	x	x			
v	vacuum, TV, stove	b	b	b	ju vacuum		
p	pipe, apples, cup	x	x	x	aɪ pipe		
b	book, baby, bathtub	x	x	x	ʊ book		
m	monkey, hammer, comb	x	x	x	o comb		SCORE
w-hw	witch, flowers, whistle	x	x	w	ɪ witch		
	I						Sounds
ð	this, that, feathers, bathe	d	v	v			I Tongue_____
h-ŋ	hanger, hanger, swing	x	ɡ	ɡ			II Lip _____
j	yes, thank you	x	x				III Vowels_____
ʒ	measure, beige	x	dʒ		ɔɪ boy		Total _____
	(story)				ɝ-ɚ bird		

Appendix IA

THE Grammatical Closure Subtest of the Illinois Test of Psycholinguistic Abilities is utilized to assess the child's expressive use of morphological structures. When dialect appropriate utterances are considered errors, the reader can clearly understand how a student can be inappropriately labeled as language delayed.

Appendix IA

ITPA Grammatical Closure Subtest and Scores *

1. Here is a dog. Here are two *dogs*.
2. This cat is under the chair. Where is the cat? She is *on* the chair.
3. Each child has a ball. This is hers, and this is *his*. (his'n)
4. This dog likes to bark. Here he is *barking*.
5. Here is a dress. Here are two *dresses*.
6. The boy is opening the gate. Here the gate has been *opened*.
7. There is milk in this glass. It is a glass *of milk*.
8. This bicycle belongs to John. Whose bicycle is it? It is *John's*.
9. This boy is writing something. This is what he *wrote*. (writed)
10. This is the man's home, and this is where he works. Here he is going to work, and here he is going *home*. (at home)
11. Here it is night, and here it is morning. He goes to work first thing in the morning, and he goes home first thing *at night*. (of the night)
12. This man is painting. He is a *painter*. (a painting;)
13. The boy is going to eat all the cookies. Now all the cookies have been *eaten*. (ate)
14. He wanted another cookie, but there weren't *any more*. (none)
15. This horse is not big. This horse is big. This horse is even *bigger*. (more bigger)
16. And this horse is the very *biggest*. (most biggest)
17. Here is a man. Here are two *men*. (mans)
18. This man is planting a tree. Here the tree has been *planted*.
19. This is soap, and these are *soap*. (soaps)
20. This child has lots of blocks. This child has even *more*.
21. And this child has the *most*. (mostest)
22. Here is a foot. Here are two *feet*. (foots)
23. Here is a sheep. Here are lots of *sheep*. (sheeps)
24. This cookie is not very good. This cookie is good. This cookie is even *better*. (gooder)

Note: The responses in parentheses were given by an Appalachian dialect speaking second grade student.

Scores:	STANDARD NORMS	LOCAL NORMS
Raw Score	9	33
Psycholinguistic Age Norm	4-8	10-4

25. And this cookie is the very *best*. (goodest)
26. This man is hanging the picture. Here the picture has been *hung*. (hanged)
27. The thief is stealing the jewels. These are the jewels that he *stole*. (stealed)
28. Here is a woman. Here are two *women*. (womans)
29. The boy had two bananas. He gave one away and he kept one for *himself*. (hisself)
30. Here is a leaf. Here are two *leaves*. (leafs)
31. Here is a child. Here are three *children*. (childrens)
32. Here is a mouse. Here are two *mice*. (mouses)
33. These children all fell down. He hurt himself, and she hurt herself. They all hurt *themselves*. (theirself)

Appendix IA

ITPA Grammatical Closure Subtest and Scores *

1. Here is a dog. Here are two *dogs*.
2. This cat is under the chair. Where is the cat? She is *on* the chair.
3. Each child has a ball. This is hers, and this is *his*.
4. This dog likes to bark. Here he is *barking*.
5. Here is a dress. Here are two *dresses*. (dress)
6. The boy is opening the gate. Here the gate has been *opened*. (open)
7. There is milk in this glass. It is a glass *of milk*.
8. This bicycle belongs to John. Whose bicycle is it? It is *John's*. (John)
9. This boy is writing something. This is what he *wrote*. (writed)
10. This is the man's home, and this is where he works. Here he is going *home*.
11. Here it is night, and here it is morning. He goes to work first thing in the morning, and he goes home first thing *at night*.
12. This man is painting. He is a *painter*.
13. The boy is going to eat all the cookies. Now all the cookies have been *eaten*. (ate)
14. He wanted another cookie, but there weren't *any more*. (none)
15. This horse is not big. This horse is big. This horse is even *bigger*. (more bigger)
16. And this horse is the very *biggest*. (most biggest)
17. Here is a man. Here are two *men*. (man)
18. This man is planting a tree. Here the tree has been *planted*.
19. This is soap, and these are *soap*. (soaps)
20. This child has lots of blocks. This child has even *more*.
21. And this child has the *most*. (mostest)
22. Here is a foot. Here are two *feet*. (foot)
23. Here is a sheep. Here are lots of *sheep*. (sheeps)

---

* *Note:* The responses in parentheses were given by a black dialect speaking first grade student.

Scores:	STANDARD NORMS	LOCAL NORMS
Raw Score	10	33
Psycholinguistic Age Norm	4-10	10-4

24. This cookie is not very good. This cookie is good. This cookie is even *better.* (gooder)
25. And this cookie is the very *best.* (goodest)
26. This man is hanging the picture. Here the picture has been *hung.* (hanged)
27. The thief is stealing the jewels. These are the jewels that he *stole.* (stold)
28. Here is a woman. Here are two *women.* (womans)
29. The boy had two bananas. He gave one away and he kept one for *himself.* (hisself)
30. Here is a leaf. Here are two *leaves.* (leafs)
31. Here is a child. Here are three *children.* (childrens)
32. Here is a mouse. Here are two *mice.* (mouses)
33. These children all fell down. He hurt himself, and she hurt herself. They all hurt *themselves.* (theirself)

Appendix IA

SENTENCE repetition tasks are used for assessment of the individual's receptive and expressive knowledge of morphology and syntax. The pathologist must have a complete understanding of dialect usage within the local community.

The following two examples illustrate standard English utterances with the corresponding dialect equivalent. Scores indicate number of correct utterances.

Without dialect consideration, test results can lead to false assumptions by the pathologist about the child's linguistic abilities causing inappropriate diagnostic labeling and inappropriate remedial placement.

Appendix IA

Sentence Repetition Test

1. He got tied up. (He got tie up.)*
2. He was washed. (He be washed.)
3. He isn't a good boy. (He ain't a good boy.)
4. Are you nice?
5. He'll be good. (He be good.)
6. Here is the toothpaste. (Here is de toofpas.)
7. Where are you going? (Where are you goin?)
8. Don't use my dough. (Do not use my dough.)
9. There isn't any more. (There ain't no more.)
10. He took it off.
11. I've got a lollipop. (I have got a lollipop.)
12. He is not going. (He ain't goin.)
13. I've already been there. (I already been there.)
14. I did read the book. (I done read de book.)
15. I'm writing daddy's name. (I writing daddy's name.)
16. I cut myself.
17. Peter is here and you are there. (Peter be here and you be dere.)
18. I see a red book and a blue book.
19. I'll give it to you if you want it. (I give it to you if you want it.)
20. He saw him so he hit him.
21. He'll eat it because its good. (He eat it because it good.)
22. David saw the bicycle and he was happy. (David saw de bicycle and he be happy.)
23. I have a pink dog.
24. I don't know what he's doing. (I do not know what he do.)
25. I want to play.
26. I like painting. (I like paintin.)
27. You have to drink milk to grow strong.
28. She does the shopping and the cooking and the baking. (She do the shoppin and the cookin and the bakin.)
29. The baby carriage is here. (The baby carriage be here.)

Standard English Score   8
Black English Score   29

---

*The sentences in the parentheses are the Black English equivalent responses.

Appendix IA

Sentence Repetition Test

1. He got tied up.
2. He was washed.
3. He isn't a good boy. (He ain't no good boy.)*
4. Are you nice?
5. He'll be good. (He be good.)
6. Here is the toothpaste.
7. Where are you going? (Where you be a'goin?)
8. Don't use my dough.
9. There isn't any more. (There ain't no more.)
10. He took it off.
11. I've got a lollipop. (I got a lollipop.)
12. He is not going. (He ain't a'goin.)
13. I've already been there. (I already been there.)
14. I did read the book.
15. I'm writing daddy's name. (I a'writin daddy's name.)
16. I cut myself.
17. Peter is here and you are there.
18. I see a red book and a blue book.
19. I'll give it to you if you want it. (I give it to you if you want it.)
20. He saw him so he hit him.
21. He'll eat it because its good. (He will eat it because its good.)
22. David saw the bicycle and he was happy.
23. I have a pink dog.
24. I don't know what he's doing. (I don't know what he's a'doin.)
25. I want to play.
26. I like painting. (I like paintin.)
27. You have to drink milk to grow strong.
28. She does the shopping and the cooking and the baking. (She does the shoppin and the cookin and the bakin.)
29. The baby carriage is here.

Standard English Score   16
Appalachian Dialect Score   29

---

*The sentences in the parentheses are the Appalachian dialect equivalent responses.

Appendix IB

B. CLINIC SAMPLES

THE first two diagnostic reports are traditionally considered to be most satisfactory, however, the reader should be aware that they are evaluations of culturally different children. No mention is given for the need to learn standard English nor of bidialectal programs to teach standard English.

The third diagnostic report is written to reflect culture and dialect considerations. Bidialectal programming to teach standard English is included in the recommendations.

RE: Sally M. Smith
Parent: Nancy Smith
Date of Birth: 10/2/79   Age: 3-10
Date of Evaluation: 8/15/83

History:

Sally was referred for this evaluation by Ms. Jane Jones, Director for Day Care Child Care Services. Mrs. Smith accompanied her daughter to this speech and language evaluation at the Speech and Hearing Clinic and indicated that her daughter would be beginning a headstart program in the fall of this year.

Medical records indicate that Sally was born between the 35th and 36th week of gestation with birthweight of 5 lbs. 5 oz. Apgar scores were eight and nine at one and five minutes after birth respectively. Sally's health has been good.

Mrs. Smith reported that developmental milestones for motor, language, and speech skills were accomplished within normal limits, she further commented that she did not believe Sally had a speech or language problem.

Significant Findings:

Sally was co-operative throughout the evaluation.

The Peabody Picture Vocabulary Test, Revised Form L yielded a receptive vocabulary age of 2-7 placing her at the third percentile and indicating development to be at the lower end of normal limits. The Preschool Language Scale yielded an auditory comprehension age of three years six months. The verbal ability subtest yielded an age equivalent of three years one and one-half months.

The Photo Articulation Test revealed substitutions for sounds which occur later maturationally, including /r,z,th,*th*,v/ and blends. A conversational sample yielded phoneme errors identical to those on the Photo Articulation Test as well as inconsistent omission of /s/ in blends and w substitution in /1/ blends.

An oral-peripheral examination revealed adequate structures for speech and language performance.

Summary:

Sally presents delayed receptive vocabulary development.

Recommendations:

1. Hearing evaluation upon entrance to Head Start.
2. Language therapy in Head Start to increase receptive vocabulary skills.

RE: Sam B. Brown
Parent: Nora Brown
Date of Birth: 4/15/80   Age: 3-3
Date of Evaluation: 7/15/83

History:

Sam was referred for this evaluation by Ms. Jane Jones, Director for Day Care Child Care Services. Mrs. Brown accompanied her son to this speech and language evaluation at the Speech and Hearing Clinic. She reported that Sam was a full term baby delivered by Caesarean Section with birthweight of 6 lbs. 9 oz. Apgar scores were four and eight at one and five minutes after birth, respectively. Medical records indicate that Sam developed pneumonia shortly after birth and was placed in the Intensive Care Nursery. Sam's health has been good.

Mrs. Brown reported that developmental milestones for motor, language and speech skills were accomplished within normal limits. She further commented that she did not believe Sam had a speech or language problem.

Significant Findings:

Sam was co-operative throughout the evaluation.

The Peabody Picture Vocabulary Test, Revised Form L, yielded a receptive vocabulary age of 2-10 placing him at the 30th percentile and indicating development to be at the low average range of normal ranking. The Preschool Language Scale yielded an auditory comprehension age of three years nine months. The verbal ability subtest yielded an age equivalent of three years nine months.

The Photo Articulation Test revealed /w/ substitutions for /l/ and /r/ blends and /t/ substitutions for the voiceless th. These consonant sounds develop at approximately the 6½ - 7½ year age range according to norms for phonological acquisition. Therefore, Sam's articulation was considered appropriate for his chronological age. Conversation sample revealed errors identical to those on the Photo Articulation Test.

An oral-peripheral examination revealed adequate structures for speech and language performance.

Summary:

Sam presents adequate receptive and expressive language skills for his chronological age. Articulation skills are also appropriate for his chronological age.

Recommendations:

No specific speech or language intervention is indicated at this time.

RE: Kendra Roberts
Parent: Martha Roberts
Data of Birth: 9/18/79 Age: 4-1
Date of Evaluation: 10/6/83

History:

Kendra was referred for this evaluation by Ms. Jane Jones, Director for Day Care Child Care Services. Ms. Roberts accompanied her daughter to this speech and language evaluation at the Day Care Center and indicated that her daughter would be enrolled in Head Start for the remainder of the year. She reported that Kendra was a full term baby with birthweight of 7 lbs. 4 oz. Kendra's health has been good.

Ms. Roberts reported that developmental milestones for motor, speech and language were accomplished within normal limits. She commented that she did not believe that her daughter had a speech or language problem.

Significant Findings:

The Photo Articulation Test revealed inconsistent omission of /s/ in blends and substitutions for /sh,ch,1,j,hw,r,th,*th*/. The latter two are characteristic of black dialect and the former ones occur later in maturation. Conversation sample revealed sound errors identical to those found in the Photo Articulation Test.

Structure and functioning of the articulators were judged adequate for speech production.

The Peabody Picture Vocabulary Test Form L yielded a receptive vocabulary age of 3-0 indicating a significant delay in understanding meaning of words.

Grammatic Closure Subtest of the Illinois Test of Psycholinguistic Abilities yielded age appropriate abilities in the area of morphology with dialect usage taken into consideration.

Expressive language sample revealed a mean length of utterance of 4.5 words. Utterances were appropriate for Black Dialect.

Summary:

Kendra presents a delay in receptive vocabulary development. Articulation errors involve sounds which occur later maturationally.

Recommendations:

1. Language therapy in Head Start to increase receptive vocabulary.
2. Bidialectal teaching of Standard English during regular class periods.
3. Parent education in bidialectal approach to teaching Standard English.

Appendix II

DO'S AND DON'TS FOR TEACHERS IN MULTICULTURAL SETTINGS*

Do's

1. Do use the same scientific approach to gain background information on the culture of multiethnic groups as you would to tackle a complicated course in science, mathematics, or any subject area in which you might be deficient.
2. Do engage in systematic study of the disciplines that provide insight into the cultural heritage, political struggle, contributions, and present-day problems of minority groups.
3. Do try to develop sincere personal relationships with minorities. You can't teach strangers! Don't give up because one black or other minority person rejects your efforts. All groups have sincere individuals who welcome honest, warm relationships with members of another race. Seek out those who will accept or tolerate you. This coping skill is one that minorities have always used.
4. Do recognize that there are often more differences within a group than between two groups. If we recognize diversity among races, we must also recognize diversity within groups.
5. Do remember that there are many ways to gain insight into a group. Visit their churches, homes, and communities; read widely and listen to various segments of the group.

---

*Cheyney, A. B., *Teaching Children of Different Cultures in the Classroom,* Columbus, Ohio: Charles E. Merrill Publishing Company, 35-37, (1976).

6. Do remember that no one approach and no one answer will assist you in meeting the educational needs of all children in a multicultural society.
7. Do select instructional materials that are accurate and free of stereotypes.
8. Do remember that there is a positive relationship between teacher expectation and academic progress.
9. Do provide an opportunity for minority group boys and girls and children from the mainstream to interact in a positive intellectual setting on a continuous basis.
10. Do provide some structure and direction to children who have unstructured lives, primarily children of the poor.
11. Do expose all children to a wide variety of literature as a part of your cultural sensitivity program.
12. Do remember that in spite of the fact that ethnic groups often share many common problems, their specific needs are diverse.
13. Do utilize the rich resources within your own classroom among various cultural groups.
14. Do remember that human understanding is a lifetime endeavor. You must continue to study and provide meaningful experiences for your children.
15. Do remember to be honest with yourself. If you can't adjust to children from multicultural homes, get out of the classroom.

Don'ts

1. Don't rely opon elementary school textbooks, teachers' guides, and brief essays to become informed on minorities. Research and resources will be needed.
2. Don't use ignorance as an excuse for not having any insight into the problems and culture of Blacks, Chicanos, Native Americans, Puerto Ricans, Asian Americans, and other minorities.
3. Don't rely on the "expert" judgment of one minority person for the answer to all the complicated racial and social problems of his/her people. For example, Blacks, Mexicans, Indians, and Puerto Ricans hold various political views on all issues.
4. Don't be fooled by popular slogans and propaganda intended to raise the national consciousness of an oppressed people.
5. Don't get carried away with the "save the world concept." Most minorities have their own savior.

6. Don't be afraid to learn from those who are more familiar with the mores and cultures than you.
7. Don't assume that you have all the answers for solving the other man's problems. It is almost impossible for an outsider to be an expert on the culture of another group.
8. Don't assume that all minority group children are culturally deprived.
9. Don't develop a fatalistic attitude about the progress of minority group pupils.
10. Don't resegregate pupils through tracking and ability grouping gimmicks.
11. Don't give up when minority group pupils seem to hate school.
12. Don't assume that minorities are the only pupils who should have multicultural instructional materials. Children in the mainstream can be culturally deprived in terms of their knowledge and understanding of other people and their own heritage.
13. Don't go around asking parents and children personal questions in the name of research. Why must they divulge their suffering? It is obvious.
14. Don't get hung up on grade designation when sharing literature that provides insight into the cultural heritage of a people.
15. Don't try to be cool by using the vernacular of a particular racial group.
16. Don't make minority children feel ashamed of their language.

Appendix III

SUGGESTIONS FOR INTERVIEWING CHILDREN*

Useful Suggestions

1. Before interviewing the child, ask the teacher or parent about areas of conversation that might stimulate the child and be related to his or her personal orientation (e.g., a pet, toys, a favorite television show, cultural holidays, his or her birthday, vacation). Use these as starters or work around them.
2. Use materials suitable to the age or level of functioning of the child. For example, for preschoolers, actual toys usually produce more speech than pictures of toys. Toys that have moving parts, as well as at least one broken toy, are good stimulus materials. In general books, toys, and brightly colored pictures are especially useful for kindergarten and elementary school children.
3. Consider the physical characteristics of the situation. It should lend itself to a naturalistic interaction rather than a structured situation such as two interactors seated formally at a table.
4. Present the child with a few items and allow for freedom of selection. When the child has made a choice, watch what he or she does with it and use the activity as a basis for conversation. If the child does not talk, make general statements such as "I won-

*Erickson, J. G., Omark, D. R., *Communication Assessment of the Bilingual Bicultural Child.* Baltimore: University Park Press, 286-289 (1981).

der what's happening", "What does it make you think of?" "I'm interested in your story about the picture." Avoid questions such as "Do you want to (or can you) tell me about that picture?" for which the child has the right to answer "No."

5. If statements or questions produce no response to stimulus items, demonstrate what you require of the child. For example, take a toy yourself and play with it, telling about what you are doing and personalize your account using an imaginary situation. Engage the child in the game as soon as possible and begin to prompt indirectly (e.g., make your car crash into the child's car and ask what happens next).

6. When the child chooses a picture and does not respond to questions, demonstrate how to talk about the picture (e.g., "This is a bad rabbit who ran away from home. He forgot to take any clothes or food with him. Luckily these two children found him and looked after him. Here's another picture. You tell me about this one."). If you have any indication of the child's language comprehension, suit your input to a level that you are confident he or she can follow, keeping in mind that if it is too simplistic you will be providing a model of what you expect from the child.

7. If you show a series of pictures depicting a sequence and then require the child to tell you the story, remove the pictures while he or she tells the story, since this will reflect a more integrated account from the child's viewpoint.

8. Vary the situation. Try to obtain a sample with the child playing a game such as keeping house, then building something, then playing with toys, etc. Interview indoors and outdoors and at the child's home when possible.

9. Vary the listener/interaction. It might be helpful to interview two children at the same time and encourage peer interaction. Observe the child with a parent or sibling and, if possible, obtain a sample from home while the child is engaged in some activity with a family member during the daily routine.

10. Record what you say (or other interviewers say) as well as what the child says in order to evaluate the utterances as related to another speaker. With these data one can gain insight into the child's comprehension as well as conversational skills.

11. Combine tape recording an interview with writing down the child's utterances as accurately as possible. In some instances it

also may be helpful to echo the child so there are no questions later when transcribing from tape. Keeping verbal (on tape) or written notes as to items or situations that stimulated the child's utterances will also be helpful.

Problems to Avoid

1. Avoid asking very specific questions that elicit yes/no answers or questions typically resulting in one word responses.
2. Avoid asking the child to tell a very familiar story that is known by heart or involves a lot of repetition of sentences.
3. Be aware of the limitations of your stimulus materials as far as vocabulary and syntax are concerned. For example, a doll house limits the child to furniture vocabulary, action pictures limit the child to the present progressive tense.
4. Modify your statements so they do not lock the response set. For example, asking, "What is he doing?" will probably elicit gerund form responses; questioning may only give you samples of declaratives and not allow the child to demonstrate the use of interrogatives; conversation related to materials present may never allow an opportunity for the child to generate past tense markers; talking about single items limits the potential use of plural markers.
5. Realize that reinforcement techniques could condition the child to produce stereotypic and repetitious responses.
6. Do not present only boy-like or girl-like toys or pictures, but allow for choice in that children will vary in their interest and background or experience.
7. Do not be concerned by silences to the point of filling in the gaps with your own verbal output. The focus is on obtaining a language sample of the child rather than that of the interviewer.

Appendix IV

TEACHER IN-SERVICE
TRAINING GUIDE

THE following outline is a guide to be used by the speech-language pathologist when instituting a bidialectal approach to teaching standard English. Plan several training sessions with teachers using a small section of the outline for each session. For example, during the first session plan to use part I, The Culturally Different and Poor Child. Experience has shown that a discussion format allowing for questions or expression of opinions is more effective than the traditional lecture format.

Appendix IV

TEACHER IN-SERVICE
TRAINING GUIDE

I. Culturally different and poor child
    A. Social characteristics
        1. Socioeconomic factors
        2. Stratification systems
        3. Sociolinguistic factors
    B. Cultural characteristics
        1. Cultural difference
        2. Cultural pluralism
        3. Cultural adaptation
II. Rationale for intervention
    A. Education
        1. Influence of dialect on academic acquisition
        2. Influence of facility with standard English
        3. Influence of current litigation and education
    B. Employability
        1. Influence of dialect
        2. Influence of listener perceptions
        3. Influence of job and social class mobility
III. Teaching methods of standard English
    A. Eradicationism
        1. Pros and cons
        2. Current research
        3. Teaching results
    B. Laissez Faire
        1. Pros and cons
        2. Current research
        3. Teaching results
    C. Bidialectalism
        1. Pros and cons
        2. Current research
IV. Role of the speech-language pathologist
    A. Culture fair assessment of speech and language disorders

   B. Culture fair treatment of speech and language disorders
   C. Bidialectal program consultant
V. Bidialectal Method
   A. Contrastive Analysis
   B. Presentation of sample lesson plans
   C. Teacher generated lesson plans*

---

*During the last in-service training session, teachers should bring regular lesson plans with them to the training session. Utilizing the bidialectal method, teachers will incorporate contrastive analysis techniques into the already existing lesson plan. In this manner teachers can learn the ease of incorporating standard English instruction in all curriculum areas.

Appendix V

SAMPLE LESSON PLANS

A. PRESCHOOL AND KINDERGARTEN

Purpose: Introduce spatial relationship words: in, over, under, and behind. Compare and contrast standard English vocabulary word "bag" with Appalachian dialect word "poke."

Materials: Large paper bag, toy car, doll, airplane, truck, and ball

Vocabulary to be contrasted:

School talk: Bag   Home talk: Poke

Sentences to be contrasted:

School Talk	Home Talk
The truck is in the bag.	The truck is in the poke.
The ball is behind the bag.	The ball is behind the poke.
The airplane is over the bag.	The airplane is over the poke.
The car is in the bag.	The car is in the poke.
The doll is under the bag.	The doll is under the poke.

Procedure:

1. Presentation of sentences:
   Compare and contrast standard English and Appalachian English versions.
   Example: The truck is in the bag.   The truck is in the poke.
2. Discrimination:
   Example: Teacher - The truck is in   Student - Different
   the bag.

		The truck is in the poke.			
Teacher	-	The doll is under the bag.	Student	-	Same
		The doll is under the bag.			

3. Identification:
    Example: Teacher - The truck is in   Student - School talk
                         the bag.
                         The truck is in   Student - Home talk
4. Translation: the poke.
    Example: Teacher - The truck is in the bag.
             Student - The truck is in the poke.
             Teacher - The doll is under the poke.
             Student - The doll is under the bag.
5. Response:
    Example: Teacher - The truck is over the poke.
             Student - No, it ain't.
             Teacher - The doll is in the bag.
             Student - No, it isn't.

In this lesson plan the target skill is learning spatial relationship words. With a very slight alteration in the regular curriculum plan, the bidialectal method is introduced at the same time. Note that through repetition of the bidialectal teaching format the target skill is acquired by the child.

A. PRESCHOOL AND KINDERGARTEN

Purpose: Introduce present progressive tense. Compare and contrast standard English and dialect forms.

Materials: Ideal Action Picture Cards

Vocabulary to be contrasted:

School Talk	Home Talk
is walking	be a walkin
is running	be a runnin
is sitting	be a sittin
is sleeping	be a sleepin

Sentences to be contrasted:

School Talk	Home Talk
He is walking.	He be a walkin.
She is running.	She be a runnin.
He is sitting.	He be a sittin.
He is sleeping.	He be a sleepin.

Procedure:

1. Presentation of sentences:
   Example: Teacher - He is walking.   He be a walking.
2. Discrimination:
   Example: Teacher - He is walking.   Student - Different
   He be a walkin.
   Teacher - She is running.   Student - Same
   She is running.
3. Identification:
   Example: Teacher - He is walking.   Student - School talk
   Student - He be a walkin.   Student - Home talk
4. Translation:
   Example: Teacher - He is walking.   Student - School talk
   Student - He be a walkin.   Student - Home talk
   Teacher - She be a runnin.
   Student - She is running.
5. Response:
   Example: Teacher - She be a walkin.
   Student - No, she ain't.
   Teacher - She is sleeping.
   Student - No, she isn't.

A. PRESCHOOL AND KINDERGARTEN

Purpose: Introduce [s] ending to quantity nouns.
Materials: Toy objects or pictures
Vocabulary to be contrasted:

School Talk	Home Talk
Balls	Ball
Blocks	Block
Dogs	Dog
Pencils	Pencil

Procedure:

1. Presentation of sentences:

    Example: Teacher - John has two balls. | John has two ball.

    Sue found three pencils. | Sue found three pencil.

2. Discrimination:

    Example: Teacher - John has two balls.
    John has two ball. | Student - Different

    Teacher - Sue found three pencil.
    Sue found three pencil. | Student - Same

3. Identification:

    Example: Teacher - Five blocks fell down. | Student - School talk
    Five block fell down. | Home talk

4. Translation:

    Example: Teacher - John has two balls.
    Student - John has two ball.
    Teacher - Two dog play.
    Student - Two dogs play.

5. Response:

    Example: Teacher - John has three ball.
    Student - No, he don't.
    Teacher - John has two balls.
    Student - Yes, he does.

B. ELEMENTARY READING:
INTRODUCTOIN OF DIAGRAPH /TH/

Utilizing a story from the basal reader, the students with teacher assistance are introduced to the new vocabulary words containing /TH/.

Vocabulary to be contrasted: mouth, birthday, bath, toothbrush, thirteen, mother, father, brother

School Talk	Home Talk
mouth	mouf
birthday	birfday
bath	baf
toothbrush	toofbrush
thirteen	firteen
mother	modder
father	fadder
brother	brodder

Sentences to be contrasted:

School Talk	Home Talk
Today is Joe's birthday.	Today is Joe's birfday.
He is thirteen years old.	He is firteen years old.
He has to take a bath.	He has to take a baf.
He lost the toothbrush.	He lost the toofbrush.
Joe's mother baked a cake.	Joe's modder baked a cake.
Joe's father bought a present.	Joe's fadder bought a present.
Joe's brother ate some cake.	Joe's brodder ate some cake.

Procedure:

1. Presentation of sentences:
   Example: Teacher - Today is Joe's birthday.   Today is Joe's birfday.

2. Discrimination:
   Example: Teacher - Today is Joe's birthday.   Student - Different
   Today is Joe's birfday.

   Teacher - He has to take a bath.   Student - Same
   He has to take a bath.

3. Identification:
   Example: Teacher - Today is Joe's Student - School talk
   birthday.
   Today is Joe's   Home talk
   birfday.

4. Translation:
   Example: Teacher - Today is Joe's birthday.
   Student - Today is Joe's birfday.
   Teacher - He has to take a baf.
   Student - He has to take a bath.

5. Response:
   Example: Teacher - Joe's fadder baked a cake.
   Student - No, he don't.
   Teacher - Joe's father bought a present.
   Student - Yes, he did.

B. ELEMENTARY READING

Purpose: Appropriate use of is and are.
Materials: "Tall Tina" by Murial Stanek*
Sentences to be contrasted:

School Talk	Home Talk
Here it is.	Here it be.
You are too tall for that seat.	You be too tall for that seat.
You are too big to cry.	You be too big to cry.
Tina is a string bean.	Tina be a string bean.
My mother is waiting for me.	My mother be waitin for me.

Procedure:

1. Presentation of sentences:
   Example: Teacher - Here it is.   Here it be.
2. Discrimination:
   Example: Teacher - Here it is.   Student - Different
                        Here it be.
            Teacher - Tina is a string Student - Same
                        bean.
                        Tina is a string
                        bean.
3. Identification:
   Example: Teacher - Here it is.   Student - School talk
                        Here it be.   Home talk
4. Translation:
   Example: Teacher - Here it is.
            Student - Here it be.
            Teacher - Tina be a string bean.
            Student - Tina is a string bean.
5. Response:
   Example: Teacher - You be too tall for that seat.
            Student - Yes, she be too tall.
            Teacher - My mother is waiting for me.
            Student - Yes, she is waiting for me.

*Short story taken from: Adams, J., *Stand Tall*, Macmillan Publishing Co., Inc., New York, 64-81, (1975).

B. ELEMENTARY READING

Purpose: Appropriate use of [s] with regular plural nouns.
Materials: "Dick Thompson the Selfish Boy" by Betty MacDonald*
Sentences to be contrasted:

Standard: 1. No one is going to touch my things.
            2. I want you to share them with your friends.
            3. He let the children look at his peppermint sticks.
            4. Inside were many locks of different sizes.

Nonstandard: 1. No one is goin to touch my thing.
            2. I want you to share them with your friend.
            3. He let the children look at his peppermint stick.
            4. Inside were many lock of different size.

Precedure:

1. Presentation of sentences:
   Example: Teacher - Inside were many locks of different sizes.
                       Inside were many lock of different size.

2. Discrimination:
   Example: Teacher - No one is going to touch my things.
                       No one is going to touch my thing.
             Student - Different
             Teacher - He let the children look at his peppermint stick.
                       He let the children look at his peppermint stick.
             Student - Same

3. Identification:
   Example: Teacher - He let the children look at his things.
                       He let the children look at his thing.
             Student - School talk
                       Home talk

4. Translation:
   Example: Teacher - Inside were many locks of different sizes.
            Student - Inside were many lock of different size.
           Teacher - He let the children look at his peppermint stick.

---

*Short story taken from: *A Second Look*, Macmillan Publishing Co., Inc. New York, 96-123, (1975).

Student - He let the children look at his pepper-
            mint sticks.

5. Response:
   Example: Teacher - No one is going to touch my things.
            Student - Yes, no one is going to touch my things.
            Teacher - There were many locks of different sizes.
            Student - Yes, there were many locks of different
                        sizes.

C. JUNIOR HIGH, HIGH SCHOOL,
AND COLLEGE LEVEL

Classroom teachers remark that dialect interferes with spelling, pronunciation, and written composition skills. These areas effect otherwise intelligent students to make poor grades in English. Teachers believe more time should be spent in the classroom improving grammar, spelling, and oral communication skills of their students. These teachers believe the students must learn standard English in order to realize the best educational opportunities available to them. The following set of lesson plans is an attempt to satisfy these needs.

Purpose: Correct oral pronunciation and written use of Where and Were.

Materials: Paper and pencil

Sentences to be contrasted:

Standard	Non-standard
Where are you going?	Were are you goin?
The books were on the shelf.	The books where on the shelf.
Where is the key?	Were is the key?

Procedure:

1. Presentation of sentences:
   Example: Teacher - Where are you going? Were are you goin?

2. Discrimination:
   Example: Teacher - Where are you going? Student - Different
   Were are you goin?

   Teacher - Where is the key? Student - Same
   Where is the key?

3. Identification:
   Example: Teacher - Where are you going? Student - Standard
   Were are you goin? Non-standard

4. Translation:
   Example: Teacher - Where are you going?
   Student - Were are you goin?

5. Response:

Example: Teacher - Were are you goin?
Student - I be a goin home.
Teacher - Where are you going?
Student - I am going home.

C. JUNIOR HIGH, HIGH SCHOOL,
AND COLLEGE LEVEL

Purpose: Correct oral pronunciation and written use of Have to vs.
Hafta.

Materials: Paper and pencil*

Sentences to be contrasted:

Standard	Non-standard
We have to go home.	We hafta go home.
They have to pay the bill.	They hafta pay the bill.
John and Jim have to work.	John and Jim hafta work.

Procedure:

1. Presentation of sentences:
   Example: Teacher - We have to go We hafta go home.
   home.

2. Discrimination:
   Example: Teacher - We have to go Student - Different
   home.
   We hafta go
   home.

   Teacher - They have to Student - Same
   pay the bill.
   They have to
   pay the bill.

3. Identification:
   Example: Teacher - We have to go Student - Standard
   home.
   We hafta go   Non-
   home.   standard

4. Translation:
   Example: Teacher - They have to pay the bill.
   Student - They hafta pay the bill.
   Teacher - John and Jim hafta work.
   Student - John and Jim have to work.

5. Response:
   Example: Teacher - We have to go home.
   Student - Yes, you do.
   Teacher - John and Jim hafta work.
   Student - Yes, them needs to work.

---

*This procedure should be done orally and then in written form.

C. JUNIOR HIGH, HIGH SCHOOL, AND COLLEGE LEVEL

Purpose: Identify dialect used in literature, its function, and identification of the standard English counterpart.

Materials: "As Ye Sow, So Shall Ye Reap," by Jesse Stewart*

Sentences to be contrasted:

Non-standard	Standard
He done his work fast.	He did his work fast.
Them books are yourn.	Those books are yours.
I didn't have no pencil.	I don't have a pencil.
They kept it for theirselfs.	They kept it for themselves.

Procedure:

1. Presentation of sentences:
   Example: Teacher - He did his work fast.   He done his work fast.

2. Discrimination:
   Example: Teacher - He did his work fast. He done his work fast.   Student - Different

   Teacher - Them books are yourn. Them books are yourn.   Student - Same

3. Identification:
   Example: Teacher - Them books are yourn. Those books are yours.   Student - Non-standard / Standard

4. Translation:
   Example: Teacher - Them books are yourn.
   Student - Yes, they be mine.
   Teacher - He did his work fast.
   Student - Yes, he did.

---

*Jesse Stewart wrote many short stories about the Kentucky mountain life. Literature is an excellent vehicle for students to learn of other cultures and dialects.

C. JUNIOR HIGH, HIGH SCHOOL, AND COLLEGE LEVEL

The following six areas can be utilized in the language arts program or English classroom.

1. Teaching dialect distinctions among language dialects and idiolect.
2. Exploring the use of dialect in literature.
3. Training students to develop their own linguistic map of their city or state.
4. Teaching the history of the English languge.
5. Studying dialects of class members without social judgment.
6. Learning the heritage of various dialects.

Using the six areas the teacher can convey the power and use of dialect within the English speaking community. Standard English skills can be taught via comparing and contrasting the dialect used by the student.

Literature:

Mark Twain uses dialect as a class caste determiner in his portrayal of Huck Finn and Jim. Students while reading can note the dialect differences used by these characters. Charles Dickens's *Great Expectations,* and Hardy's *Mayor of Casterbridge* also are rich in the use of dialect that students can compare and contrast during class discussion about the literature.

Pragmatics:

In less structured setting, students need practice in using standard English appropriately in a manner that is meaningful to them. The following list suggests ways to facilitate pragmatic usage in the classroom.

1. News Interview: One student sits in the front of the class. Class members question the student about his life history, interests, and opinions about relevant issues. One group of students verbalize in dialect while one group is required to use standard English. The student being interviewed must give a dialect response to a dialect question and a standard English response to a standard English question.
2. Group Story: Each member of the class contributes a sen-

tence to a story. Once the story has been written the class as a whole makes corrections so that the final form is written in standard English.

3. Journal Writing: Ten minutes of class time per week are used for independent writing in standard English on any topic the student desires.

4. Correction of Journal Writing projects are done by the class as a whole.

5. Cartoons without captions: First orally and then in writing students create the dialogue for each frame of a cartoon in standard English.

6. Students make up television commercials both orally and in written form utilizing standard English.

7. Skits: Place six to ten objects in a paper bag. Divide the students into small groups giving each group a bag of objects. Students are to generate a story situation with the objects and present the skit to the class in standard English.